oxygen's

ROBERT KENNEDY'S
WOMEN'S FITNESS

PICK*it*
KICK*it*

SIMPLE CHOICES, HUGE RESULTS

Diane Hart

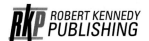

RKP *ROBERT KENNEDY*
PUBLISHING

Published by Robert Kennedy Publishing
400 Matheson Blvd. West
Mississauga, ON
L5R 3M1 Canada
Visit us at www.rkpubs.com
www.pickitkickit.com

Managing Senior Production Editor: Wendy Morley
Online and Associate Editor: Vinita Persaud
Junior Production Editor: Cali Hoffman
Art Director: Gabriella Caruso Marques
Acting Art Director: Jessica Pensabene
Editorial Designer: Brian Ross
Assistant Editor: Stephanie Maus
Proofread by: Karen Petty
Indexing: James De Medeiros

Library and Archives Canada Cataloguing in Publication

Hart, Diane,
    Oxygen's Pick it, kick it : simple choices, huge results / by Diane Hart.

ISBN 978-1-55210-075-2

    1. Diet. 2. Nutrition. 3. Food habits. 4. Reducing diets. 5. Weight loss.
6. Reducing diets--Recipes. I. Title. II. Title: Pick it, kick it.

RM222.2.H364 2010   613.2'5   C2010-901368-9

10 9 8 7 6 5 4 3 2 1

Distributed in Canada by
NBN (National Book Network)
67 Mowat Avenue, Suite 241
Toronto, ON
M6K 3E3

Distributed in USA by
NBN (National Book Network)
15200 NBN Way
Blue Ridge Summit, PA
17214

Printed in Canada

IMPORTANT

The information in this book reflects the author's experiences and opinions and is not intended to replace medical advice.

Before beginning this or any nutritional or exercise regimen, consult your physician to be sure it is appropriate for you. Ask for a physical stress test.

This book is dedicated to the many *Oxygen* readers who generously shared their inspirational personal stories of fat loss and continue to motivate others in their quest to live the *Oxygen* lifestyle.

Contents ● ● ●

INTRO 6

1. **BREAKFAST: SLASH CALORIES WITHOUT EVEN TRYING!** ... 8
Quick and easy combos; breakfast building blocks.

2. **LUNCH: LEAN UP YOUR LUNCH!** Is your salad ... 42
making you fat? salad bar guide; be soup savvy.

3. **DINNER: EASY DINNERTIME FAT LOSS.** ... 92
Simple dinners for gals on the go; time-saving tips
for you; importance of mindful eating.

4. **SNACKS: GO AHEAD, HAVE A SNACK!** (In fact, have a few!) ... 142
Filling snacks; portion control.

5. **EATING OUT – HOW TO GRAB A BITE WITHOUT
PACKING ON THE POUNDS.** BONUS! Your fast-food guide: ... 176
how to get what you want; your restaurant survival guide;
favorite pick it / kick its for pizza, sushi and burgers.

6. **IN YOUR CUPBOARD: SHAPE UP YOUR KITCHEN.** ... 206
Stock your shelves with staples. BONUS! Excerpt from
Clean Eating magazine on three pantry must-haves;
bust fat with your groceries; pantry checklist; label lingo;
everyday foods that blast fat.

7. **GOOD-FOR-YOU FOODS: EAT BETTER FEEL BETTER.** ... 248
10 ways to get more energy from your food; nutrients to
keep you lean; the right kind of fat; the wrong kind of fat;
food for better sleep. BONUS! How to kick the salt habit.

8. **EXCLUSIVE PICK IT RECIPES** ... 312

HOW TO USE THIS BOOK

All too often, weight loss appears overwhelming. Those last 10 pounds may seem impossible to lose. But *Pick it Kick it* makes it easy (really) to shed flab. Take a look below to see your guide to the book – at every meal and snack you have the opportunity to make tiny changes and reap big benefits!

 It's all about making smarter choices. This plan is your perfect guide!

Your Game Plan

(our step-by-step guide to the easiest weight you'll ever lose!)

If you want to LOSE FAT

FINALLY lose pounds for good!

How to eat mindfully to drop a dress size! **118**

Top 15 ways to shed flab without even noticing! **226**

Your restaurant survival guide **196**

BONUS! Fast-food guide! **178**

PLUS! Your best and worst menu picks! **202**

8 calorie-cutting tips to drop pounds easily **160**

Bust fat with your groceries: a guide to healthy shopping **210**

If you want to EAT RIGHT

Foods you want to eat that are easy and no fuss. Hello, fat loss!

Find healthy meals you'll love! Need a menu makeover for every meal of the day?

Breakfast 8

BONUS! Your guide to the best oats! 31

Lunch 42

Is your salad making you fat? 54

Dinner 92

Slurp your way slim with soup! 86

Snacks 144

If you want to
GET MOTIVATED

Everyday women share their real-life secrets to weight loss.

"I switched from white pasta to whole wheat pasta!" **40**

"I always order a sweet potato at a restaurant – plain, of course!" **90**

"I always snack on air-popped popcorn, raw veggies or rice cakes!" **140**

"I use small whole wheat tortillas instead of bread for sandwiches!" **174**

"I completely ditched the sugary sodas. Now I drink green tea and water, water, water!" **204**

"I snack on roasted red pepper hummus with sliced carrots instead of baked chips with dip!" **246**

"I always grill instead of fry!" **310**

If you want to
STAY ON TRACK

Once you lose the weight, you need to know how to keep it off.

Nutrients to keep you lean **276**

The right kinds of fats.
PLUS! The wrong kinds of fats! **277**

A guide to portions **209**

Stock your shelves with the best stay-slim foods **208**

BONUS! Your 3 pantry must-haves! **208**

If you want to
STAY HEALTHY

Get lean, get energized and stay that way for the rest of your life.

Eat better to feel better **250**

10 ways to get more energy from your food. PLUS! 5 top energy snacks! **296**

Shake your salt habit! **252**

BONUS! Your 3-day low-sodium meal plan **257**

PICK IT! RECIPES

Drop pounds with the best weapon... our fat-fighting recipes!

Two minutes to your best homemade dressing **56**

You must try these sandwiches! **68**

Ditch fat-laden recipes and lose the pounds, not the taste! **312**

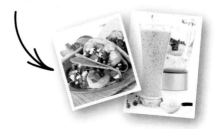

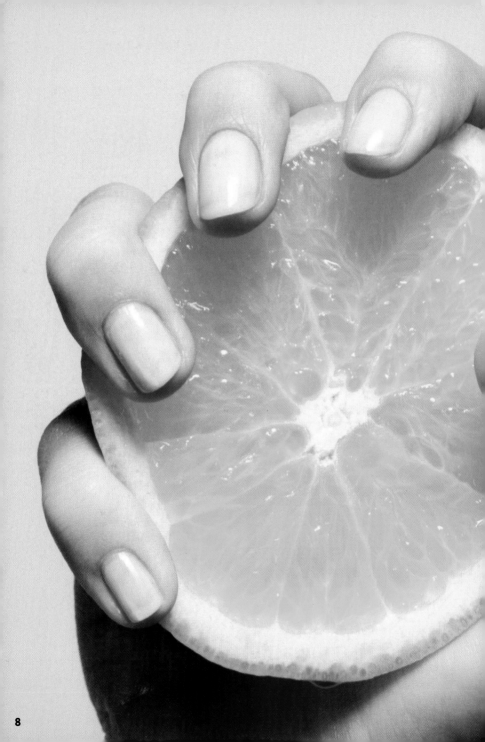

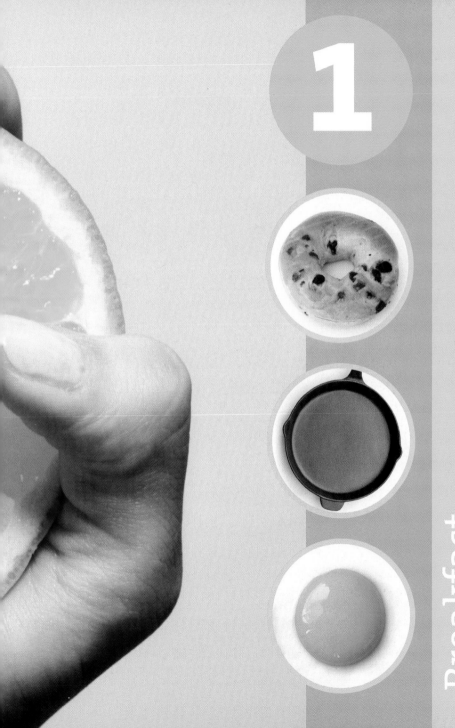

1

Breakfast

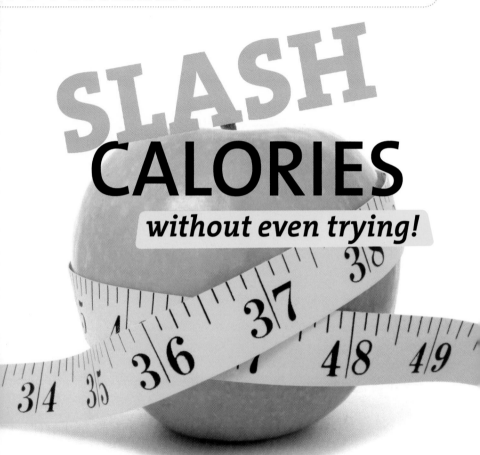

SLASH CALORIES

without even trying!

I may just be the only person in the world who insists on purchasing eyeliner based on one single requirement – that it can be applied at red lights during the morning commute. So you can see that for me – likely for you too – a healthy, nutritious breakfast has to be no-fuss at the very least. Plus, fast and portable. And yet I realize that if I skip breakfast, as do almost 30 percent of Americans, I run the risk of watching my waist get bigger and my dress size larger. Plus, I'm cranky at my desk by mid-morning. Research increasingly links skipping breakfast with long-lasting weight gain. Breakfast stokes your metabolic furnace throughout your busy day and keeps weight gain at bay.

Like so many things that can make a difference, it's all about making smarter choices. And they don't have to be difficult. It may be nice to sit down to eggs, whole wheat toast, orange juice and coffee, but when you're digging your pumps out of the closet, grabbing your phone, dropping the kids off at school and then facing the morning commute, you will likely just grab what's easiest: a bagel and cream cheese, weighing in at a hefty 450 calories, or a breakfast sandwich at the local café, at almost 500 calories. Switch it up and you'll save calories without even trying.

Research has shown that if you lose weight, you'll keep it off by eating breakfast. Recent findings from the National Weight Control Registry (a group of more than 5,000 people who have lost a minimum of 30 lbs and kept them off for at least a year), 78 percent said they ate breakfast every day while 90 percent said they ate it four times a week. Other research found dieters who ate a protein-rich breakfast lost more weight in eight months than those who didn't eat something rich in protein. Protein in your first meal of the day is critical. A 2008 study published in the *British Journal of Nutrition* noted that if you add extra protein into your breakfast – some egg whites, a piece of meat, even a scoop of almond butter in oatmeal – you'll feel fuller throughout the day.

So the message is clear – eat a good breakfast (and find a make-up gal you trust to recommend only the easiest-to-apply eyeliner).

Q&A

Q *I don't want to eat breakfast before my early morning workout because I am concerned I will not burn fat during my weight training. What would be a good pre-workout snack?* -Emily

A I understand your concern about eating a full breakfast prior to a morning workout, but think about your body like a race car. If there's no fuel in the tank, it won't run well. All night your body is fasting, which means you have depleted your glycogen (stored carbohydrates) reserves by morning.

Complex carbohydrates such as whole grain breads and oatmeal will replenish glycogen stores. Some suggestions include a whole grain bagel with natural peanut butter, low-fat mozzarella string cheese with an apple or steel-cut oatmeal with a tablespoon of ground flaxseed – yummy!

TOP TIP: To build strength, make sure to consume enough nutrients (300 to 400 extra calories per day) to keep up with your training sessions.

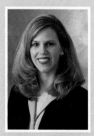

AMY JAMIESON-PETONIC, M.Ed., RD, ADA Spokesperson and Employee Wellness Manager at the Cleveland Clinic.

PICK IT

Nutritional Value

SERVING	1 Tbsp
CALORIES	29
FAT	0 g
CARBS	7.3 g
FIBER	0.3 g
SUGAR	6 g
SODIUM	3 mg
PROTEIN	0 g

Apple Butter

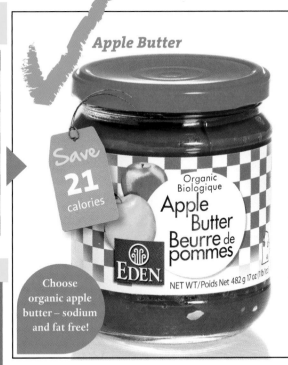

Save
21
calories

Organic
Biologique

Apple
Butter
Beurre de
pommes

EDEN

NET WT/Poids Net 482 g 17 oz (1 lb 1 oz)

Choose organic apple butter – sodium and fat free!

BONUS!

Fruits and vegetables

contribute dietary nutrients that combat inflammation, thus reducing the risk of heart disease, cancer and other chronic illnesses. A daily glass of orange juice boosts "good" HDL cholesterol to help keep arteries from becoming clogged, and it's a good source of potassium to help lower risk of high blood pressure and stroke. Dairy products add the calcium necessary for strong bones, and many prepared cereals are fortified with folate (to combat birth defects) and other important vitamins and minerals.

Give It a Try!

Low-cal fruit spread (1 tsp)
8 calories, 0 fat, 2 g carbs

All natural organic honey (1 tsp)
19 calories, 0 fat, 5.2 g carbs

Two large strawberries, sliced
12 calories, 0.1 g fat, 2 g carbs

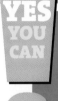

YES
YOU
CAN

Buddy up. Grab a friend and make a date for an early-morning workout. You can burn up to 350 calories!

12

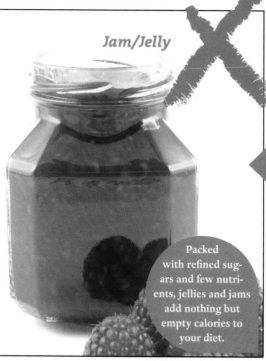

Jam/Jelly

Packed with refined sugars and few nutrients, jellies and jams add nothing but empty calories to your diet.

KICK IT

Nutritional Value	
SERVING	1 Tbsp
CALORIES	50
FAT	0 g
CARBS	13 g
FIBER	0 g
SUGAR	12 g
SODIUM	0 mg
PROTEIN	0 g

MAKE IT BETTER

Spread peanut butter on whole wheat toast or a wrap. Add half an apple or banana for a crunchy or sweet lunch.

Ditch These Too!

Regular orange marmalade (1 Tbsp)
49 calories, 0 fat, 13.3 g sugar

Concord grape jelly (1 Tbsp)
50 calories, 0 fat, 13 g sugar

Lemon curd (1 Tbsp)
60 calories, 1 g fat, 11 g sugar

35

The size of a woman's waist, in inches, which puts her at an increased risk of developing metabolic syndrome. To stave off belly fat, add whole grains to your diet.

— American Heart Association

Say What?

STUDIES SHOW that eating breakfast is the key to weight loss, productivity and upping your energy levels. "When people skip breakfast, they set themselves up for overeating at the end of the day and gaining weight," says Nancy Clark, MS, RD, sports nutritionist and author of *Nancy Clark's Sports Nutrition Guidebook* (Human Kinetics, 2008).

PICK IT

Nutritional Value	
SERVING	1
CALORIES	290
FAT	12 g
CARBS	30 g
FIBER	2 g
SUGAR	3 g
SODIUM	760 mg
PROTEIN	16 g

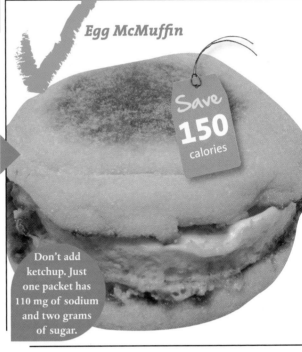

Egg McMuffin

Save **150** calories

A BETTER CHOICE

Order two scrambled eggs with one slice of whole wheat toast.

Don't add ketchup. Just one packet has 110 mg of sodium and two grams of sugar.

Give It a Try!

Plain English muffin with trans-fat-free margarine
180 calories, 3 g fat, 300 mg sodium

McDonald's Breakfast Burrito
300 calories, 16 g fat, 7 g saturated fat, 2 g sugar, 830 mg sodium

McDonald's Fruit and Yogurt Parfait (with granola)
160 calories, 2 g fat, 85 mg sodium, 150 mg calcium

TOP CHOICE! *Green Tea*

Not only will this traditional Asian brew help you chill out, drinking green tea will also give you an added fat-burning boost. A new study by Korean researchers found that green tea extract reduces fat tissue, which means you may also reap the same benefits from a supplement form. According to L.A. based nutritionist Jennifer Stoynev, RD, green tea can also increase your energy and decrease your cholesterol.

BREW IT
Steep a batch, then add lemon and ice, and chill. This makes a great twist on traditional iced tea.

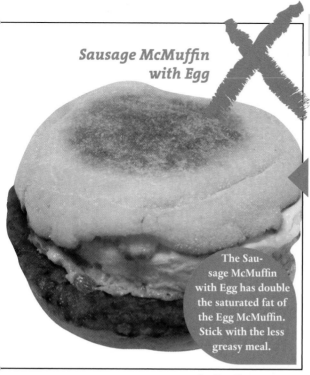

Sausage McMuffin with Egg

Nutritional Value	
SERVING	1
CALORIES	440
FAT	26 g
CARBS	32 g
FIBER	2 g
SUGAR	2 g
SODIUM	980 mg
PROTEIN	21 g

The Sausage McMuffin with Egg has double the saturated fat of the Egg McMuffin. Stick with the less greasy meal.

INSTANT MEAL COMBO

One whole grain English muffin with two Tbsp peanut or almond butter.

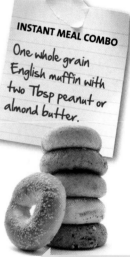

Ditch These Too!

McDonald's Hotcakes with syrup
530 calories, 9 g fat, 46 g sugar

McDonald's Big Breakfast
740 calories, 48 g fat, 1,560 mg sodium

Bacon and egg bagel
530 calories, 18 g fat, 1,370 mg sodium

BONUS!

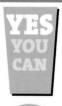

YES YOU CAN

Ditch caffeine. When paired with cortisol – the stress hormone – caffeinated drinks will become fat's best friend, helping your body hang on to it. Dump that extra cuppa joe!

Whole grain toast, muffins, waffles and bagels provide a good base to your meal by contributing carbohydrates and fiber.

PICK IT

Oatmeal

Save 138 calories

Nutritional Value	
SERVING	1 cup
CALORIES	147
FAT	2.3 g
CARBS	25.3 g
FIBER	4 g
SUGAR	0.6 g
SODIUM	2 mg
PROTEIN	6.1 g

DON'T LIKE OATMEAL? Replace it with any whole grain hot cereal with less than five grams of sugar and more than three grams of fiber.

Give It A Try!

☑ **Nature's Path Flax Plus granola (multi-bran)**
250 calories, 9 g fat, 36 g carbs

☑ **Whole Foods Shredded Wheat (not frosted)**
170 calories, 1 g fat, 40 g carbs

☑ **Red River Cereal**
154 calories, 2.5 g fat, 27 g carbs

INSTANT MEAL COMBO *Oatmeal topped with a sprinkle of brown sugar and walnut halves, plus a half-cup of strawberries.*

TOP CHOICE!
Cinnamon

Research has found that cinnamon may reduce blood glucose concentrations after your meal. So spicing it up in a variety of dishes will help you burn fat! Cinnamon helps control insulin levels (so it discourages fat storing and encourages fat burning) and has clinically proven anti-microbial properties (it helps to stop the growth of bacteria).

ALTHOUGH HIGH IN VITAMINS B12 AND B6, GRANOLA IS ALSO HIGH IN SUGAR.

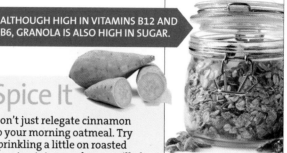

Spice It

Don't just relegate cinnamon to your morning oatmeal. Try sprinkling a little on roasted sweet potatoes and even grilled chicken for an unexpected flavor burst that also blasts fat.

Cook your own oatmeal and you'll cut out the extra sugar contained in many instant pre-packaged varieties. Serve with a half-cup of skim milk (adds calcium), and top with a half-ounce of chopped nuts (for protein and healthy fat) and half of a chopped apple or sliced banana (vitamin C and potassium). You'll get a slimming, but filling, 340-calorie meal with 12 grams of protein and 7 grams of fiber.

Nutritional Value

SERVING	½ cup
CALORIES	285
FAT	3.8 g
CARBS	60 g
FIBER	4.5 g
SUGAR	21 g
SODIUM	165 mg
PROTEIN	6 g

Ditch These Too!

✕ **Kellogg's Frosted Mini-Wheats (bite size)**
200 calories, 1 g fat, 30 g carbs

✕ **Post Just Bunches**
250 calories, 7 g fat, 43 g carbs

✕ **Muesli cereal**
289 calories, 4 g fat, 66 g carbs

MAKE IT BETTER

Add cinnamon for flavor, sweetness and a host of other benefits.

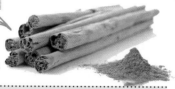

SAY WHAT? A new study in the *Journal of Nutrition* shows that women who eat a high-fiber, low-sugar breakfast tend to burn more fat. Oatmeal, yogurt and fruit are all good picks. Eat more frequent smaller meals throughout the day to increase your metabolism. By boosting your metabolism, you'll burn more calories, even when you sleep. Hello, fat loss!

PICK IT

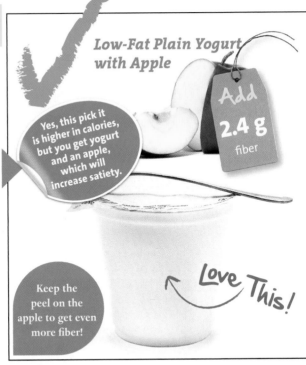

Nutritional Value

SERVING	1 cup
CALORIES	207
FAT	4.1 g
CARBS	31.1 g
FIBER	2.4 g
SUGAR	27.7 g
SODIUM	173 mg
PROTEIN	13.2 g

Low-Fat Plain Yogurt with Apple

Yes, this pick it is higher in calories, but you get yogurt and an apple, which will increase satiety.

Add **2.4 g** fiber

Keep the peel on the apple to get even more fiber!

Love This!

EVEN BETTER

Swap out sugar-packed, nutrient-bereft cereals for yogurt and strawberries, and you'll trick your body into feeling fuller. The reason? When protein is digested, it causes the release of CCK, the hormone that makes you feel full.

Give It a Try!

Stoneyfield Farms organic fat-free plain yogurt
80 calories, 0 fat, 12 g carbs

Trader Joe's nonfat Greek style yogurt – honey, blueberry or pomegranate
150 calories, 0 fat, 16 g carbs

Dannon Light & Fit Carb & Sugar Control smoothie (7 fl oz)
60 calories, 2.5 g fat, 3 g sugars, 4 g carbs

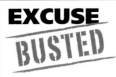

EXCUSE
BUSTED

I hate dieting, it leaves me hungry all day.

Eating clean allows you to eat five or six meals a day, and will leave you fuller and more energized than your previous diet.

MAKE IT **BETTER**

- Top with fresh raspberries or blueberries and a crunchy whole grain cereal.
- Look for fortified plain yogurt for more nutrients.

KICK IT

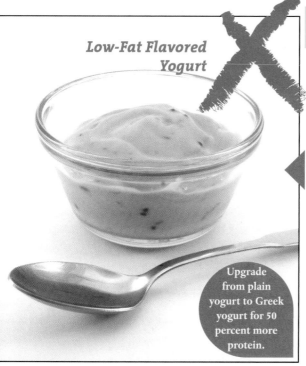

Low-Fat Flavored Yogurt

Nutritional Value	
SERVING	1 cup
CALORIES	174
FAT	1.9 g
CARBS	32.5 g
FIBER	0 g
SUGAR	32.4 g
SODIUM	99 mg
PROTEIN	7.4 g

Upgrade from plain yogurt to Greek yogurt for 50 percent more protein.

Say What?

PEOPLE WHO eat breakfast are 50 percent less likely to be obese than those who don't eat breakfast.

Ditch These Too!

Fruit-on-the-bottom yogurt (6 oz)
150 calories, 1.5 g fat, 28 g carbs

Yoplait smoothie (8 oz)
220 calories, 3 g fat, 43 g carbs

X

La Crème yogurt – fruit flavour (4 oz)
*140 calories, 5 g fat,
19 g carbs, 65 mg sodium*

Try This

Pairing low-fat plain yogurt (protein) with strawberries (fruit – high water/fiber content) is a flab-free way to lose calories without losing sweetness.

BONUS!

Start your day

off right and you won't go wrong, trust me! What you eat at breakfast establishes your nutritional pattern for the whole day. A balanced breakfast should supply about one-fourth of the day's protein plus fiber-rich complex carbohydrates and a small amount of healthy fat.

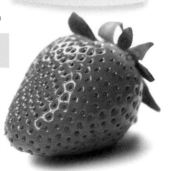

PICK IT

Nutritional Value

SERVING	2 egg whites
CALORIES	34
FAT	0.1 g
CARBS	0.5 g
FIBER	0 g
SUGAR	0.5 g
SODIUM	110 mg
PROTEIN	7.2 g

EVEN BETTER

Include protein and healthy fat in your breakfast by topping toast with baked beans, eggs, peanut butter or low-fat cheese. Scramble diced chicken or turkey with your eggs for a protein-packed punch!

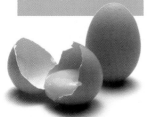

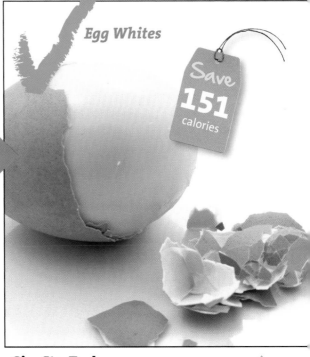

Egg Whites

Save
151
calories

Give It a Try!

Egg Beaters
30 calories, 0 fat, 1 g carbs ✓

Egg whites scrambled with mushrooms, tomatoes and peppers
45 calories, 0 fat, 112 mg sodium ✓

Two-egg-white omelet (made with a splash of milk and a sprinkle of salt and pepper)
43 calories, 0 fat, 278 mg sodium ✓

YES YOU CAN

When it comes to weight loss, stay consistent and don't get discouraged by the numbers on the scale. Don't give up – you need to use up 3,500 extra calories to lose one pound. You may notice a larger loss in your first week – this is due to a decrease in water weight from depleted glycogen stores, and decreases in sodium and carbs. After that, the body utilizes its fat and protein stores. Water and hormonal shifts also affect the number on the scale.

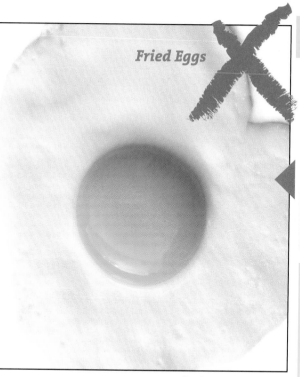
Fried Eggs

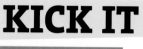

KICK IT

Nutritional Value	
SERVING	2 fried eggs
CALORIES	185
FAT	14 g
CARBS	0.8 g
FIBER	0 g
SUGAR	0.8 g
SODIUM	188 mg
PROTEIN	12.5 g

> **QUICK & EASY**

Scrambled eggs made with one whole egg and two egg whites, one cup of spinach and half a cup of chopped tomatoes, all sautéed in one Tbsp olive oil and served with two slices of whole grain toast.

Ditch These Too!

 Eggs Benedict on toast or English muffin
613 calories, 31 g fat, 59 g carbs

 Eggs Florentine on toast or English muffin
890 calories, 59 g fat, 25 g carbs

 Hash browns
207 calories, 9.8 g fat, 27.4 g carbs

Say What?

ONE WHOLE egg provides up to 15 percent of your daily value of iodine, a trace element that is essential for good thyroid function and effective metabolic function. It also helps your body utilize calcium efficiently.

ALL YOU!

GET THE POWER OF BREAKFAST WORKING FOR YOU. What's not to like about scoring big payoffs at work, school or in your relationships because your mind and body are functioning in top-notch form?

PICK IT

Shredded Wheat

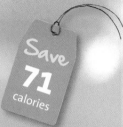

Save 71 calories

AVOID frosted shredded wheat.

Nutritional Value	
SERVING	2 biscuits
CALORIES	169
FAT	1.1 g
CARBS	39.4 g
FIBER	6 g
SUGAR	0.5 g
SODIUM	3 mg
PROTEIN	5.7 g

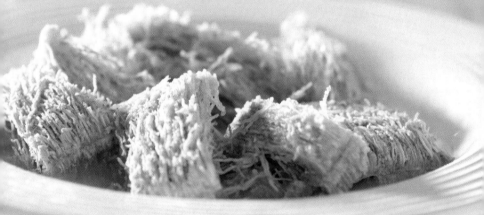

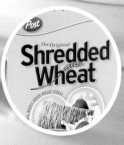

Give It A Try!

✓ **Spoon-Size Shredded Wheat (½ cup)**
85 calories, 0 sugar, 0 sodium

✓ **Grape Nuts (¼ cup)**
200 calories, 4 g sugar, 290 mg sodium

✓ **General Mills Wheaties (¾ cup)**
100 calories, 4 g sugar, 190 mg sodium

USE LOW-FAT MILK.

A CUP OF BLUEBERRIES HAS NEARLY FOUR GRAMS OF STAY-FULL FIBER!

FATTER, NOT FITTER

- High in sugar and saturated fat!
- The label says it all: brown sugar, sugar and high fructose corn syrup are all listed.

General Mills Oatmeal Crisp Almond

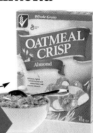

DIABETIC WOMEN who eat a diet rich in whole grains, bran and fiber significantly reduce their chance of developing heart disease.

QUICK & EASY ▼

One cup whole grain cereal with one cup skim milk and one banana.

JUST BECAUSE A CEREAL CONTAINS OATMEAL DOESN'T MEAN IT'S GOOD FOR YOU. READ THE LABEL.

TOP CHOICE!
Mixed Berries

Packed with antioxidants, blueberries and raspberries are also very low in calories. Japanese scientists have discovered that these berries also contain capsaicin, a substance that dissolves fat. Further, blueberries have 84 calories per cup and raspberries have only 64 per cup, making both excellent low-cal produce picks.

Nutritional Value

SERVING	1 cup
CALORIES	240
FAT	5 g
CARBS	46 g
FIBER	4 g
SUGAR	16 g
SODIUM	116 mg
PROTEIN	6 g

Ditch These Too! ↘

✗ **Post Banana Nut Crunch**
240 calories, 6 g fat, 12 g sugar

✗ **Special K Fruit and Yogurt (¼ cup)**
120 calories, 1 g fat, 11 g sugar

✗ **Cracklin Oat Bran (½ cup)**
200 calories, 7 g fat, 15 g sugar

Add It ≫

For a hint of natural sweetness, add half a cup of fresh berries to your cereal.

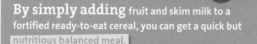

By simply adding fruit and skim milk to a fortified ready-to-eat cereal, you can get a quick but nutritious balanced meal.

PICK IT

Nutritional Value

SERVING	1 muffin
CALORIES	290
FAT	2.5 g
CARBS	62 g
FIBER	2 g
SUGAR	32 g
SODIUM	750 mg
PROTEIN	4 g

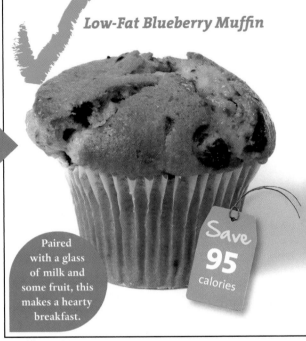

Low-Fat Blueberry Muffin

Paired with a glass of milk and some fruit, this makes a hearty breakfast.

Save **95** calories

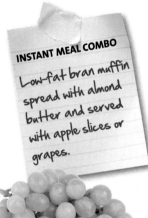

INSTANT MEAL COMBO

Low-fat bran muffin spread with almond butter and served with apple slices or grapes.

Give It a Try!

Hostess 100-calorie packs
100 calories, 3 g fat, 22 g carbs

Trader Joe's Minis – blueberry
80 calories, 1.5 g fat, 22 g carbs

Bluebran Vitamuffin
100 calories, 0 fat, 23 mg sodium

BONUS!

Boost your brain power

After sleeping all night, you have to break the fast and refuel in order to feel energetic and perform at your best. Since your brain doesn't have reserves of glucose, its main energy source, you can enhance your mental clarity by replenishing glucose with carbohydrates consumed at breakfast. The nutrients in your morning meal contribute to improved alertness, concentration, creativity, memory, mood and problem-solving ability.

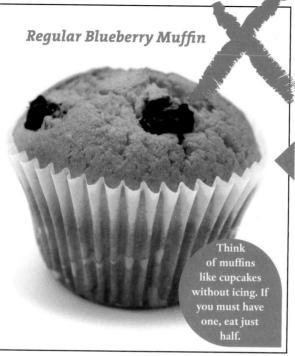

Regular Blueberry Muffin

Nutritional Value	
SERVING	1 muffin
CALORIES	385
FAT	9 g
CARBS	66.7 g
FIBER	3.6 g
SUGAR	27.4 g
SODIUM	621 mg
PROTEIN	7.6 g

Think of muffins like cupcakes without icing. If you must have one, eat just half.

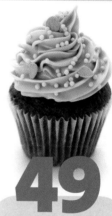

Ditch These Too!

Trader Joe's banana chocolate chip muffin
430 calories, 17 g fat, 65 g carbs

My Favorite Muffin – chocolate chip
633 calories, 33 g fat, 81 g carbs

Dunkin' Donuts coffee cake muffin
620 calories, 25 g fat, 54 g sugar, 93 g carbs, 530 mg sodium

49

Percentage of women participating in a comprehensive Harvard Medical School / Brigham and Women's Hospital study who were less likely to gain weight after consuming more fiber-rich whole grains than those who ate foods made from refined grains.

Say What?

YO-YO DIETING not only fails to keep the weight off, it can also cause heart disease, according to a study in the *International Journal of Obesity*. When it comes to creating a balanced diet, focus on whole grains, fresh produce and lean protein – for the rest of your life, not as a quick fix.

PICK IT

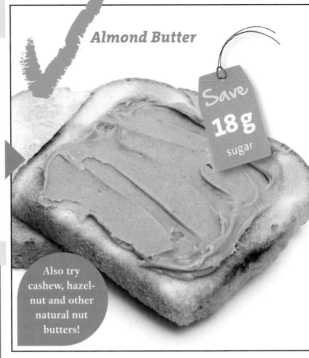

Almond Butter

Save **18 g** sugar

Also try cashew, hazelnut and other natural nut butters!

BONUS!

In 2009, Harvard researchers found that women who ate nuts at least twice per week kept their weight down over an eight-year period.

Give It a Try!

Hazelnut butter (2 Tbsp)
180 calories, 1 g sat. fat, 1 g sugar

Pistachio butter (2 Tbsp)
190 calories, 1.5 g sat. fat, 2 g sugar

Soy spread (2 Tbsp)
170 calories, 1.5 g sat. fat, 3 g sugar

TOP CHOICE! *Nuts*

Many research studies have linked nuts with increased fullness without the associated weight gain. In fact, current research published in the *Journal of Nutrition* shows that people who eat nuts more often have a reduced body fat. Overall, eating nuts in moderation will improve your chance at weight loss success. Plus, as an added health benefit, nuts will also reduce your cholesterol levels.

CRACK IT
With just one ounce of almonds you'll get about 80 grams of calcium while reducing your body fat.

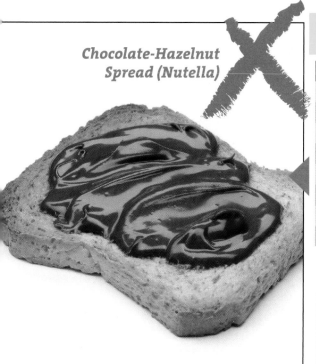

Chocolate-Hazelnut Spread (Nutella)

KICK IT

Nutritional Value	
SERVING	2 Tbsp
CALORIES	200
FAT	12 g
CARBS	22 g
FIBER	2 g
SUGAR	20 g
SODIUM	10 mg
PROTEIN	2 g

EXCUSE BUSTED

I need to eat less than 1,000 calories a day to shed pounds faster.

Jamie Larsen, RD, LD, registered dietitian for the Emily Program, an eating disorders treatment program, warns, "Consuming less than your basic caloric needs, about 1,200 calories a day for women, actually slows your metabolism and puts your body into starvation mode. In starvation mode, your body doesn't allow for weight loss."

Ditch These Too!

Chocolate cream cheese spread (2 Tbsp)
120 calories, 6 g sat. fat, 6 g sugar

Commercial peanut butter (2 Tbsp)
190 calories, 3 g sat. fat, 3 g sugar

Butter (2 Tbsp)
102 calories, 7.3 g sat. fat, 0.1 g sugar

Say What?

EATING JUST two ounces of nuts per day, such as almonds, walnuts and peanuts, lowers your LDL cholesterol by about five percent.

PICK IT

Nutritional Value	
SERVING	1 cup
CALORIES	147
FAT	2.3 g
CARBS	25.3 g
FIBER	4.3 g
SUGAR	0.6 g
SODIUM	2 mg
PROTEIN	6.1 g

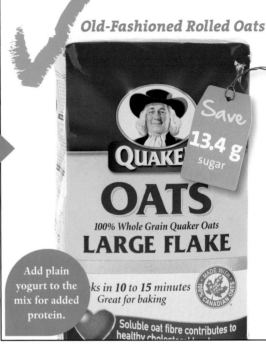

Old-Fashioned Rolled Oats

Save **13.4 g** sugar

QUAKER

OATS
100% Whole Grain Quaker Oats
LARGE FLAKE

Add plain yogurt to the mix for added protein.

...ks in **10 to 15** minutes *Great for baking*

MADE WITH 100% CANADIAN OATS

Soluble oat fibre contributes to healthy chol...

Q&A

Q *What's the difference between instant oatmeal and steel cut? Why is steel cut considered better?*

A When it comes to a nutritious, hearty breakfast, a bowl of steel-cut oatmeal is about as good as you can get. Steel-cut oats, also known as Irish or Scottish oats, have been minimally processed, which maintains their nutty flavor and chewy texture as well as their natural fiber and nutrients. Steel-cut oatmeal takes about 15 minutes to prepare (or just a few in the microwave), but the flavor is well worth it. You can also incorporate steel-cut oats into granola, oatcakes and other treats. If you have the time, steel-cut or old-fashioned oats should be your first choice.

Give It a Try!

Old-fashioned oatmeal (1 cup) with flaxseed (1 Tbsp) *202 calories, 6.3 g fat, 28.3 g carbs*

Large-flake oatmeal (1 cup) with either wheat germ or oat bran (1 Tbsp) *174 calories, 3.1 fat, 28.8 g carbs, 5.4 g fiber*

Cooked multigrain hot cereal (1 cup) *260 calories, 2 g fat, 0 sodium*

MAKE IT **BETTER**

Sprinkle a teaspoon of ground flaxseed on top of your oats to double the fiber!

Instant Oatmeal

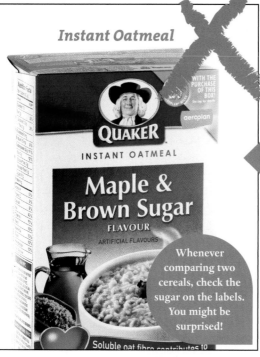

> Whenever comparing two cereals, check the sugar on the labels. You might be surprised!

KICK IT

Nutritional Value	
SERVING	1 packet
CALORIES	170
FAT	2 g
CARBS	33 g
FIBER	3 g
SUGAR	14 g
SODIUM	220 mg
PROTEIN	4 g

Say What?

REST IS key to weight loss. Sleep charges up your fat-burning system and impacts appetite-controlling hormones. Also, during deep sleep, your body releases human growth hormone (HGH), which builds and repairs muscles. Aim for eight hours of shut-eye every night.

Ditch These Too!

Flavored instant oatmeal
140 calories, 2.5 g fat, 27 g carbs

Quaker oatmeal chocolate chip breakfast cookie
180 calories, 6 g fat, 14 g sugar, 190 mg sodium

X

Instant Cream of Wheat – apples 'n cinammon (1 cup)
260 calories, 0 fat, 32 g sugar, 320 mg sodium

BONUS!

Stir unsweetened applesauce into cooked oatmeal or make bran muffins with shredded carrots to increase your daily fruit and veggie servings.

FATTER, NOT FITTER

- Flavored instant oatmeal is higher in calories and sugar!
- Add extra brown sugar to your oats and you'll double the sugar!

A Healthy Breakfast

Has at Least

5

Grams of Protein

LOW-FAT OR NONFAT DAIRY PRODUCTS CAN ADD PROTEIN to your breakfast, as can egg whites or egg substitute (egg yolk doesn't contribute protein); lean breakfast meats such as Canadian back bacon, extra-lean ham, turkey bacon or light turkey sausage; and soy milk and other soy products. Here's how much protein you get from some typical breakfast foods:

Breakfast Protein Sources	Protein (g)	Calories	Fat (g)	Saturated Fat (g)	Carbs (g)
Skim milk, 1 cup	10	100	0	0	14
Low-fat yogurt, vanilla, 1 cup	9.3	253	4.6	2.6	42
Low-fat cottage cheese, 1 cup	28	160	2	1	6
Reduced-fat cheese, 1 ounce	8	70	4	2.5	1
Stonyfield Farms organic low-fat yogurt, fruit flavored	7	110	0	0	22
Egg substitute, 1/4 cup	6	30	0	0	1
Low-fat Soy milk, 1 cup	4	90	1.5	0	14
Soy-based sausage, 2 ounces	12	119	4.5	0.7	6
Tofu, extra firm lite, 2 ounces	5	43	1.4	0	2.2
Canadian (back) bacon, 2 ounces	12	89	3.9	1.2	1
Extra lean ham, 2 ounces	11	61	1.5	0.4	0.4
Turkey bacon, 2 strips	4	70	6	1	< 1
Light turkey sausage, 2 ounces	9	130	10	2.2	1
Peanut butter, natural, 1 tablespoon	3.5	100	8	1	3.5
Light cream cheese, 1 ounce	3	53	4	2.7	1.8
Lox (smoked salmon), 1 ounce	5.2	33	1.2	0.2	0

YOUR GUIDE *to the* BEST OATS

THE MOST POTENT WEAPON YOU MAY NEED FOR your fat loss is a simple one – oats. A recent Pennsylvania State University study found that individuals on a weight-loss plan that included whole grains reduced their belly fat more than those who ate the same diet but included only refined grains. Other research showed that women who eat the most whole grains are the least likely to gain weight as they age. From a health perspective, whole grains provide greater benefits than refined grains. And according to research, individuals who eat two or more servings of whole grains daily can reduce their risk of hypertension and all cardiovascular diseases by as much as 21 percent.

WHOLE GRAIN The grain in whole grain bread, pasta and rice has the bran, germ and endosperm left intact. These contain the most beneficial antioxidants, trace minerals and natural fats. Whole grains tend to have a lower GI rating than most refined grains and offer numerous health benefits.

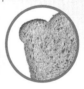

DURUM WHEAT This is the wheat used to make most pasta. When milled, the endosperm of durum is made into semolina. Pasta products will say durum semolina, semolina or whole wheat durum, or a blend of both on their ingredient lists. Since semolina is not a whole grain, look for pastas that contain whole wheat durum flour.

GLUTEN FREE This means that a food or product is free of wheat, rye, barley and for some, oats. If you have celiac disease – about one in 133 Americans have permanent adverse reactions to gluten – look for gluten-free alternatives like amaranth, arrowroot, beans, corn, millet, nut flours, potato, quinoa, rice, soy and sorghum, among others.

» KNOW YOUR OATS

Find out which oats are best for you!

OAT BRAN »

The outer layer of the oat kernel, oat bran is high in soluble fiber. Use it in baked goods and breakfast cereal.

OAT CONVERSION

½ cup raw oats = 1 cup cooked oats

ROLLED OATS »

Otherwise known as standard oatmeal and old-fashioned oats, rolled oats are whole oats that have been steamed, rolled and flaked so that they cook quickly. You can prepare them in about five to ten minutes.

QUICK OATS »

Instant oats are quick oats that have been precooked so that they only need to be mixed with hot liquid. These oats are rolled even thinner than steel-cut or rolled oats, making them less chewy and less flavorful than slower-cooking oats. While you can cook quick oats in about three to five minutes, they do not provide the long-term energy of their rolled or steel-cut cousins.

« STEEL-CUT

Oats that are whole-grain groats chopped into pieces are called steel-cut. They're chewier than rolled oats and can take 20 minutes or longer to cook.

Food	Fiber Content in Grams
Oatmeal, 1 cup	3.98
Whole wheat bread, 1 slice	2
Whole wheat spaghetti, 1 cup	6.3
Brown rice, 1 cup	3.5
Barley, 1 cup	13.6
Buckwheat, 1 cup	4.54
Rye, 1/3 cup	8.22
Corn, 1 cup	4.6
Apple, 1 medium with skin	5.0
Banana, 1 medium	4.0
Blueberries, 1 cup	3.92
Orange, 1 large	4.42
Pear, 1 large	5.02
Prunes, 1/4 cup	3.02
Strawberries, 1 cup	3.82
Raspberries, 1 cup	8.36

PICK IT

Nutritional Value	
SERVING	3 slices
CALORIES	105
FAT	9 g
CARBS	0 g
FIBER	0 g
SUGAR	0 g
SODIUM	540 mg
PROTEIN	6 g

Turkey Bacon

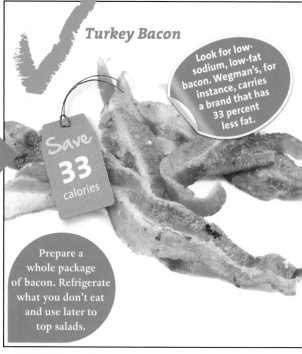

Look for low-sodium, low-fat bacon. Wegman's, for instance, carries a brand that has 33 percent less fat.

Save **33** calories

Prepare a whole package of bacon. Refrigerate what you don't eat and use later to top salads.

400 million
Number of obese adults worldwide.

MAKE IT BETTER

Snip turkey bacon into small pieces and scramble together with one whole egg and two egg whites.

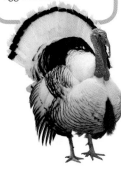

Give It a Try!

Extra lean ham
140 calories, 6.5 g fat, 0.4 g carbs

Canadian bacon
89 calories, 4 g fat, 0.7 g carbs

Tofu
117 calories, 7 g fat, 3.5 g carbs ✓

Say What?

SKIPPING MEALS doesn't make you lose weight – it makes you gain because of blood sugar fluctuations that can trigger you to reach for junk food. And if you think you're giving yourself wiggle room by starving, think again. It'll backfire on you because you'll likely rack up far more calories than you otherwise would at your next meal. Plus, you slow down your metabolism when you go too long between meals.

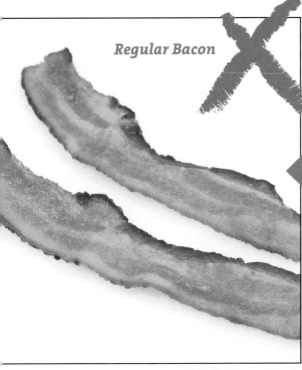

Regular Bacon

KICK IT

Nutritional Value	
SERVING	3 slices
CALORIES	138
FAT	10.7 g
CARBS	0.4 g
FIBER	0 g
SUGAR	0 g
SODIUM	589 mg
PROTEIN	9.4 g

YES YOU CAN

Eat white turkey meat instead of beef and pork whenever possible. A study in March 2009 tied excessive red meat consumption to higher risk of death from cancer and heart disease. - *Archives of Internal Medicine*

Ditch These Too!
BLT with mayonnaise
550 calories, 34 g fat, 42.5 g carbs

Bacon and fried eggs
272 calories, 20.8 g fat, 1 g carbs

Jumbo sausage
286 calories, 22.7 g fat, 3.6 g carbs

TIP Add half a grapefruit to your breakfast. A study from the *Journal of Medicinal Food* shows that grapefruit can help you lose up to ten pounds in twelve weeks along with exercise.

 FAST FACT

Take your time when you eat. Rushing while munching won't make you feel full and you'll likely snack again. Relax and chew! For more on mindful eating, go to page 118.

RECIPE ▶ **For a great recipe using turkey bacon, turn to page 71.**

PICK IT

Nutritional Value

SERVING	2 waffles
CALORIES	140
FAT	2.5 g
CARBS	27 g
FIBER	3 g
SUGAR	3 g
SODIUM	410 mg
PROTEIN	4 g

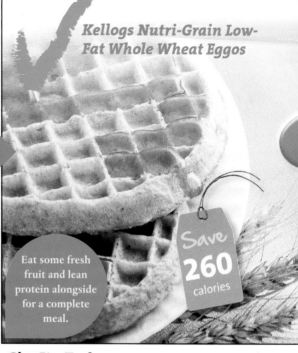

Kellogs Nutri-Grain Low-Fat Whole Wheat Eggos

Eat some fresh fruit and lean protein alongside for a complete meal.

Save **260** calories

35

Percentage of Americans who skip breakfast.

Buy protein powder in your favorite flavor and you'll satisfy your cravings without the guilt. For example, try a chocolate flavor if you're known to reach for chocolate bars.

Give It a Try!

Kashi Go Lean waffles
170 calories, 3 g fat, 4 g sugar, 330 mg sodium

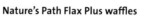

Nature's Path Flax Plus waffles
180 calories, 7 g fat, 5 g sugar, 380 mg sodium

Nature's Path buckwheat waffles with real berries
180 calories, 6 g fat, 4 g sugar, 350 mg sodium

TOP CHOICE! *Protein Shakes*

Researchers have found that protein shakes really do help people lose weight. While it's important to watch out for added sugar, getting in the extra protein will help keep your body in prime fat-loss mode. Including protein shakes in your diet will also help you lose fat because it's an effective and easy way to ensure proper portion control.

SHAKE IT
Keep your body in fat-frying mode by keeping an extra stash of protein powder in your gym bag or purse so you can stir up a quick shake when you're on the run.

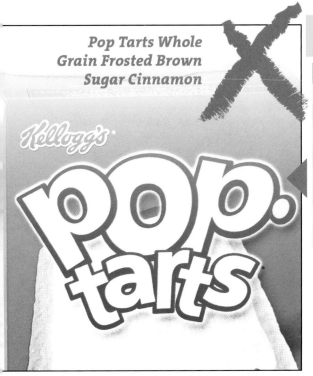

Pop Tarts Whole Grain Frosted Brown Sugar Cinnamon

Kellogg's pop. tarts

Nutritional Value	
SERVING	2 tarts
CALORIES	400
FAT	12 g
CARBS	68 g
FIBER	10 g
SUGAR	24 g
SODIUM	320 mg
PROTEIN	6 g

INSTANT MEAL COMBO

Multigrain frozen waffle topped with fresh banana slices and a hardboiled egg on the side.

Have just one waffle (or the minis) to cut calories and fat.

Ditch These Too!

Van's Belgian Homestyle waffles
172 calories, 3.5 g fat, 30 g carbs

Eggo waffles – cinnamon toast
150 calories, 5.5 g fat, 8.5 g sugar, 245 mg sodium

Pillsbury pancakes – chocolate burst
280 calories, 7 g fat, 51 g carbs

EXCUSE BUSTED

My genes won't allow me to be slim.
Refined sugar and a sedentary lifestyle won't carve out that body either. Test out some small changes – you'll be happy with the results.

54 million
Number of people in the U.S. with pre-diabetes, known as metabolic syndrome.

PICK IT

Nutritional Value	
SERVING	1
CALORIES	260
FAT	2 g
CARBS	51 g
FIBER	3 g
SUGAR	7 g
SODIUM	470 g
PROTEIN	12 g

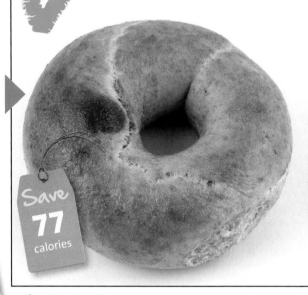

Whole Grain Bagel

Save
77
calories

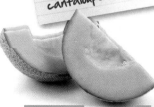

INSTANT MEAL COMBO

Whole grain bagel alongside low-fat cottage cheese and a quarter cantaloupe.

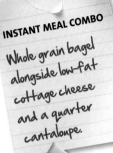

Give It a Try!
Whole wheat English muffin
130 calories, 1 g fat, 25 g carbs

Sprouted grain bagel
280 calories, 1.5 g fat, 2 g sugar, 390 mg sodium

Perfect 10 Western Bagel – healthy grain
140 calories, 2 g fat, 1 g sugar, 370 mg sodium

>> FAST FACT
Water really does speed up weight loss, according to the journal Obesity. *In one study women who drank one liter of water a day lost up to five pounds more than those who did not.*

YES YOU CAN

Figure out the truth behind the words. The only real way to tell if a food item is truly "whole" grain is to read the label. Choose only bagels that list whole grains or whole grain flour as the first ingredient.

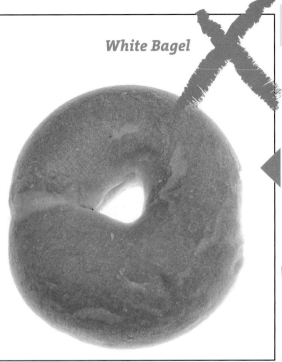

White Bagel

Nutritional Value	
SERVING	1 medium
CALORIES	337
FAT	2 g
CARBS	66 g
FIBER	3 g
SUGAR	7 g
SODIUM	587 mg
PROTEIN	13 g

YES YOU CAN Burn more energy than you consume. **Make smarter food choices and get moving – it's a winning combination.**

Ditch These Too!
Cinnamon donut
290 Calories, 18 g fat, 3 g protein

Bagel with smoked salmon and regular cream cheese
362 Calories, 9 g fat, 1,652 mg sodium, 21 g protein

Au Bon Pain – cinnamon crisp bagel
410 calories, 7 g fat, 24 g sugar, 390 mg sodium

Say What?

REGISTERED DIETITIAN and sports nutrition expert Tammy Beasley of Huntsville, Alabama, says a breakfast with three parts carbohydrate and one part protein takes a lot of energy for your body to break down and keeps you full for hours.

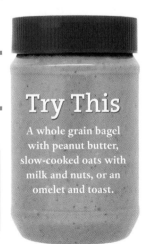

Try This

A whole grain bagel with peanut butter, slow-cooked oats with milk and nuts, or an omelet and toast.

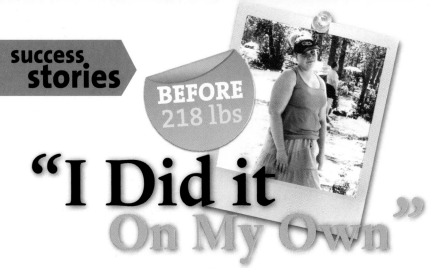

BEFORE
218 lbs

"I Did it
On My Own"

Despite a lack of support from loved ones, this classroom supervisor found an inner drive and lost almost 90 lbs.

BY ASTRID VAN DEN BROEK

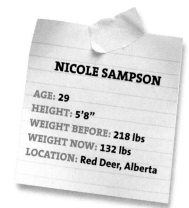

NICOLE SAMPSON

AGE: 29

HEIGHT: 5'8"

WEIGHT BEFORE: 218 lbs

WEIGHT NOW: 132 lbs

LOCATION: Red Deer, Alberta

"I just figured that eating healthy and working out would help me gain that sense of control."

GAINING CONTROL

Nicole did what experts say makes the difference between success and failure – she started with small changes when she began eating clean. She cut out "the whites"— bread, pasta and sugar — and began eating more vegetables and fruits. She also created her own home gym with 10-lb weights, bands, balls, a stair stepper and her long-neglected treadmill. "I made up my own program from reading tips in *Oxygen*," she says. Once she got into her groove, she wanted to keep going. "I used working out as a focus, as time for myself," she says. "I could think through things while on the treadmill and take out frustration on my strength-training days."

After going through a difficult breakup, Nicole Sampson wanted to take charge of a life she viewed as wildly out of control. She was in her 20s, weighed 218 lbs and was in major need of a self-esteem boost. "I just figured that eating healthy and working out would help me gain that sense of control." And with that, she began the first steps towards her new life.

ALL ON HER OWN

When she reached 150 lbs, Nicole was motivated to continue. But, with nobody cheering on her weight loss, she felt alone in her journey. "The majority of my friends and family were not always supportive of what I was doing," she says. "I heard comments such as, 'You should gain about 10 lbs back' and 'Are you eating?'" Wanting both to prove to herself that she could do it and show others that her new lifestyle was healthy, Nicole kept working hard despite the criticism.

NEWFOUND SUPPORT

Today, at 132 lbs, Nicole continues her workouts and clean-eating habits, guilt free. She realizes that her friends and family just needed some time to adjust to her new look. "They are supportive now that they're used to it," she says. And now they ask her for fat loss advice, too. With the confidence and knowledge she has gained, Nicole is just the right person to ask. "I am the person I've always wanted to be. And I did it myself."

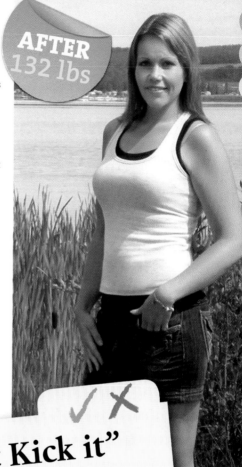

AFTER
132 lbs

"My Pick it Kick it"

BREAKFAST

PICK IT
Natural peanut butter

KICK IT
Regular peanut butter

SNACKS

PICK IT
Cottage cheese flavored with a sprinkling of seasoning

KICK IT
Dip for veggies

MY SUCCESS TIP: "I switched from white pasta to whole wheat pasta!"

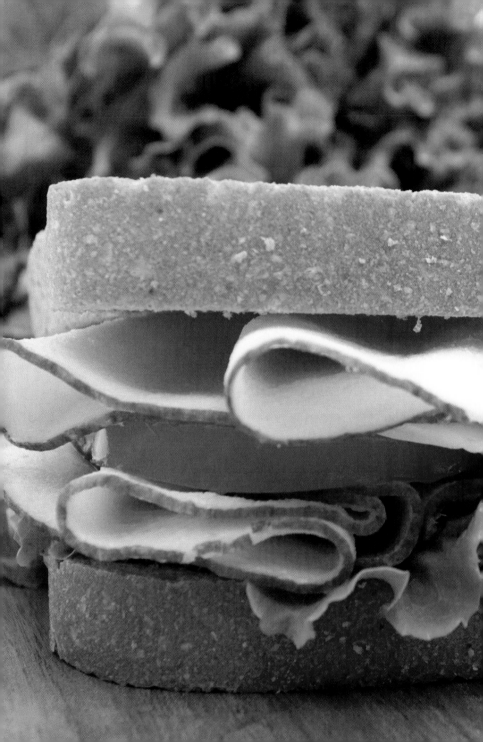

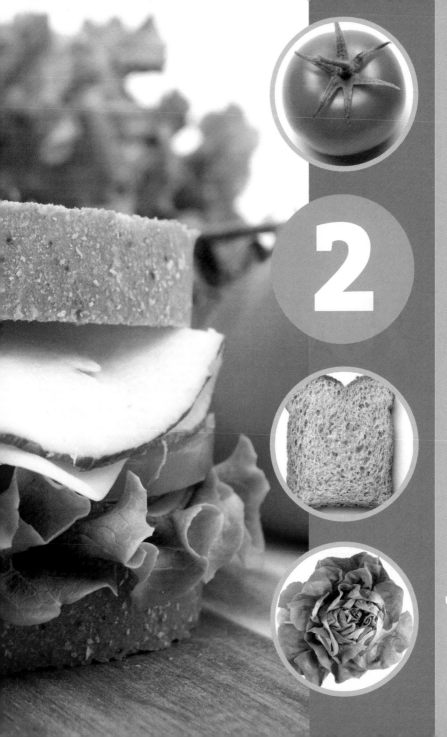

2

Lunch

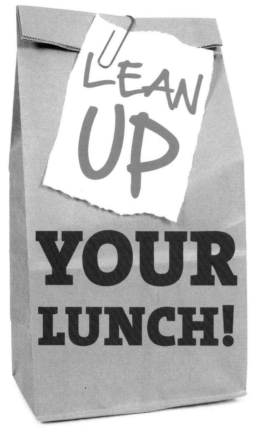

Fess up! When it comes to lunch, do you tend to eat at your desk? I know I do – too often. As much as I want to take a lunch break, the day gets away from me and I find myself munching away as I check my email or go through layouts. Not a good habit!

So what do you eat for lunch? A sensible sandwich, leftovers from last night or perhaps a light salad if you've got weight loss on your "to do" list. But these foods can be deceiving – you may assume you're saving calories when really you're packing much heavier meals that won't do a thing for your waistline, except help it expand!

A salad isn't always the smartest choice. If your leafy greens are buried under a heap of dressing, cheese, croutons and other toppings, you can wind up with a salad that has more calories and fat than a Big Mac (540 calories and 29 g of fat, 10 g of which are saturated!). Studies at Penn State University revealed that when it's prepared right (dressed with balsamic vinaigrette or a homemade vinegar-based dressing), eating a salad as a first course prevents you from overeating at your meal. The fiber and water-rich ingredients fill you up, so it feels like you're eating more without piling on tons of extra calories. The same goes for broth-based soups.

Every meal you eat should contain complex carbs from vegetables and/or grains, lean protein and healthy fats. This is the magic combo that will keep you satisfied without weighing you down. Hear that ladies? No more deprivation.

BUILD YOUR PLATE AROUND THIS VISUAL:

Vegetables and Grains
50%

Lean Protein
25%

Healthy Fats
25%

If you're serious about making healthy changes you're going to have to be aware of everything on your plate. So many women think toppings, nibbles, condiments and little bites don't make a difference … but they do! In fact, research points to a growing number of women who eat the

majority of their calories via salads. And yes, ladies, the dressings and toppings make all the difference.

For instance, croutons can be a diet downfall. They contribute saturated fat and calories with little nutritional value. If you're looking for crunch atop your greens, a much better choice is unsalted sunflower seeds that provide healthy fats and important B vitamins as well. Bacon bits? What's the point, unless you want a salt and fat overload?

The same goes for the mayonnaise in your sandwich. Mayo and other creamy dressings quickly turn healthy meals into cheeseburger deluxes – heavy on the clogged arteries. A better bet is mustard, or, if you're looking for a richer taste and feel without the added fat and calories, a thick, yogurt- or bean-based spread such as tzatziki or hummus. And beware of "light" versions. Fat free does not equal calorie free and the term "light" is relative to the original version. Even light dressings can contain up to 70 calories (or more!) per tablespoon.

Even if you have to eat at your desk, take 10 minutes to eat without reading emails, shuffling through papers or checking phone messages. Pay attention to how you feel before, during and after your meal. Make note of how hungry you are, how full you feel when you're done and again after 20 minutes (it can take this long for your brain to receive "full" signals from your stomach). When it comes to lunch, don't munch mindlessly.

PICK IT

Nutritional Value	
SERVING	200 g (with 1 Tbsp olive oil)
CALORIES	299
FAT	14 g
CARBS	41 g
FIBER	7 g
SUGAR	13 g
SODIUM	72 mg
PROTEIN	4 g

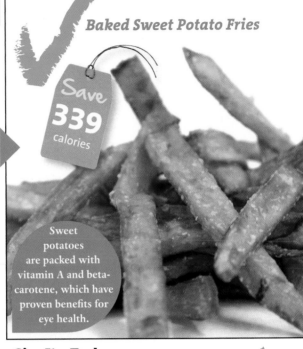

Baked Sweet Potato Fries

Save **339** calories

Sweet potatoes are packed with vitamin A and beta-carotene, which have proven benefits for eye health.

YES YOU CAN

Set your goal and stick to it. Enter a local fitness competition, half marathon or triathlon to give yourself some extra incentive. Setting goals, working toward them and seeing the progress will strengthen your independence and sense of self-worth, two crucial elements for a woman's psychological and spiritual well-being.

≫ FAST FACT

Research has shown a link between watching TV and eating more. Turn off the tube to stay lean.

Give It a Try!

Baked sweet potato fries (half portion)
149.5 calories, 7 g fat, 20.5 g carbs

Homemade fry dip (1 Tbsp salsa and ½ cup plain low-fat yogurt)
82 calories, 2 g fat, 10 g carbs

Savory sweet potato fries (1 Tbsp parmesan cheese and dried rosemary leaves)
159 calories, 4.3 g fat, 26.4 g carbs

YES YOU CAN

When it comes to potatoes, it's not what's in them (good stuff, by the way!) but what you put on them and how you cook them (bake, boil or grill 'em!). Potatoes contain high amounts of health-promoting nutrients including vitamin C, potassium and fiber (which helps to maintain the stability of heart cells and the central nervous system).

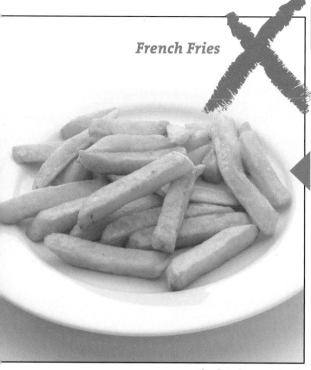

French Fries

KICK IT

Nutritional Value	
SERVING	200 g
CALORIES	638
FAT	34 g
CARBS	76 g
FIBER	8 g
SUGAR	2 g
SODIUM	388 mg
PROTEIN	8 g

Try This

Cut sweet potatoes into wedges, coat in olive oil and your favorite spices, and bake at 425°F for about 20 minutes. Turn midway through.

Ditch These Too!

Onion rings
440 calories, 21 g fat, 55 g carbs

Oven heated frozen fries
130 calories, 4 g fat, 17 g carbs

Tater tots
240 calories, 15 g fat, 24 g carbs

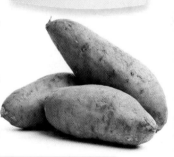

Say What?

GET RID OF YOUR DEEP FRYER! Researchers are continuing to explore the link between deep frying and carcinogernic acrylamide, a toxic element formed in carbohydrate-rich foods cooked at high temperatures such as deep frying. Additionally, compounds common to the Western diet produced by high-temperature cooking or frying are linked to increased inflammation that may lead to a higher risk of chronic diseases. Although research is still preliminary, deep frying foods such as potato chips or fries is not recommended – it adds saturated fats and unhealthy calories to your diet.

PICK IT

Nutritional Value

SERVING	½ cup
CALORIES	80
FAT	0 g
CARBS	18 g
FIBER	3 g
SUGAR	10 g
SODIUM	470 mg
PROTEIN	3 g

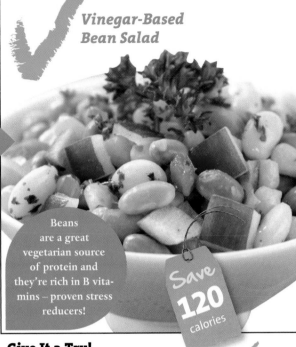

Vinegar-Based Bean Salad

Beans are a great vegetarian source of protein and they're rich in B vitamins – proven stress reducers!

Save **120** calories

EXCUSE BUSTED

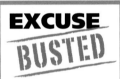

Clean, healthy food is too expensive.

Clip coupons, buy in bulk, and choose in-season fruits and veggies. Beans, oats and rice offer huge nutrition for just a few cents per serving. Make soups and stews. Have a cup of low-sodium vegetable juice before lunch – a nutritious drink that helps you eat less for just pennies a day. And make sure to sip lots of water – it's free!

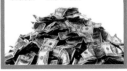

Give It a Try!

Bulgar salad
70 calories, 2 g fat, 12 g carbs

Greek salad with green beans
110 calories, 4.1 g fat, 16.9 g carbs

Corn and black bean salad
123 calories, 5.6 g fat, 14.7 g carbs

Say What?

EATING HEALTHY meals every two to three hours keeps your blood sugar and insulin levels on an even keel. Insulin spikes from irregular mealtimes (especially when you eat starches and sugars) makes you store fat, not burn it.

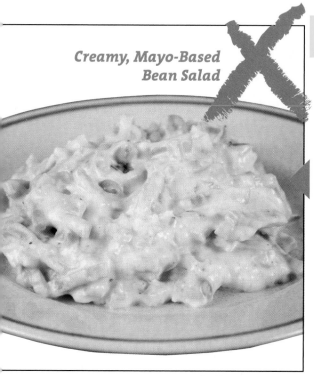

Creamy, Mayo-Based Bean Salad

KICK IT

Nutritional Value	
SERVING	½ cup
CALORIES	200
FAT	7 g
CARBS	26 g
FIBER	6 g
SUGAR	13 g
SODIUM	278 mg
PROTEIN	11 g

Try This

Want to eat beans without feeling gassy? Always make sure you soak them well in cold water and then change the water before you cook them.

Ditch These Too!

Macaroni salad
227 calories, 11.3 g fat, 25.9 g carbs

Seafood with crab and shrimp
272 calories, 19.3 g fat, 19.3 g carbs

Potato salad with mayo
200 calories, 10 g fat, 24 g carbs

▶ QUICK & EASY

Salad made with a 6-oz can of low-sodium chunk light tuna + ½ cup tinned beans + 1 ½ cups baby spinach + ½ cup chopped red peppers + 2 Tbsp honey mustard vinaigrette. Calories: 422, Total Fat: 13 g, Saturated Fat: 1 g, Trans Fat: 0 g, Cholesterol: 50 mg, Sodium: 650 mg, Carbohydrates: 37 g, Dietary Fiber: 8 g, Sugar: 6 g, Protein: 41 g

MAKE IT **BETTER**

Serve with a side of brown rice for even more lasting power!

PICK IT

Nutritional Value	
SERVING	1 salad
CALORIES	230
FAT	11 g
CARBS	12 g
FIBER	4 g
SUGAR	4 g
SODIUM	665 mg
PROTEIN	21 g

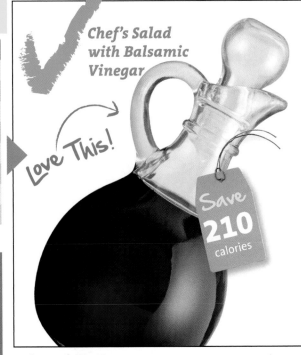

Chef's Salad with Balsamic Vinegar

Love This!

Save **210** calories

YES YOU CAN

Think yourself thin. Visualization has been proven in recent studies to aid in fat loss — "I think I'm thin, therefore I am."

BONUS!

Instead of pouring the dressing on your salad, dip the tines of your fork in the dressing and then have a bite.

TIP Nix croutons and add double cucumbers for crunch! Always order a salad with dressing on the side.

Give It a Try!
Dole Asian Crunch kit
120 calories, 6 g fat, 12 g carbs

Spinach salad with unsalted sunflower seeds
85 calories, 7 g fat, 5 g carbs

Fresh Express Salsa Ensalada! kit
120 calories, 8 g fat, 10 g carbs

Say What?

EAT FOR BETTER VISION? Researchers at Harvard Medical School and Brigham and Women's Hospital in Boston tracked 36,000 women for 10 years. Their study revealed that women who ate lots of fresh fruits and vegetables had a 10 to 15 percent less chance of contracting cataracts than those who did not eat plenty of these foods. Cataracts involve a clouding of the eye lens, leading to blurred vision and eventually blindness.

Chef's Salad with Thousand Island Dressing (2 oz)

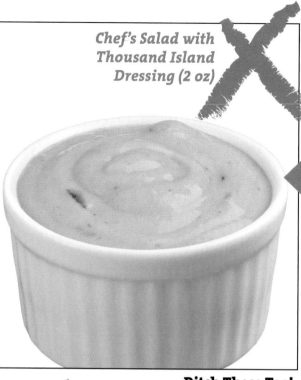

KICK IT

Nutritional Value	
SERVING	1 salad
CALORIES	440
FAT	30.9 g
CARBS	20.1 g
FIBER	4.5 g
SUGAR	12.6 g
SODIUM	1,154 mg
PROTEIN	21.6 g

PACK IT
TO GO

Stay fit and frugal with these lunchtime must-haves: sturdy aluminum containers and a water canteen to keep you safe from harmful plastic toxins – all packed in our very own insulated bag, which is a surefire way to remind yourself to eat clean, stay hydrated and train hard!

Oxygen cooler - $19.95; shopmusclemag.com.

Ditch These Too!

Chef's salad with regular ranch dressing
375 calories, 26.4 g fat, 14 g carbs

Garden vegetable salad with peppercorn ranch dressing
360 calories, 34 g fat, 10 g carbs

Mexican taco salad with salsa
600 calories, 31 g fat, 56 g carbs

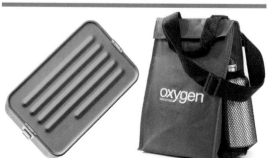

PICK IT

Nutritional Value

SERVING	1 salad
CALORIES	85
FAT	7 g
CARBS	5 g
FIBER	2 g
SUGAR	1 g
SODIUM	36 mg
PROTEIN	4 g

 FAST FACT

Nuts and sunflower seeds contain Omega-6 fatty acids. According to a recent advisory from the American Heart Association, this EFA can reduce your risk of heart disease.

BONUS!

Although

higher in calories and fat, sunflower seeds are a better choice than croutons because they contain mono- and polyunsaturated fats. This means they're going to keep you full and help protect your heart.

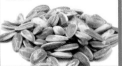

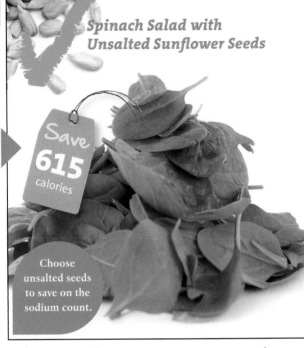

Spinach Salad with Unsalted Sunflower Seeds

Save **615** calories

Choose unsalted seeds to save on the sodium count.

Give It a Try!

Balsamic vinaigrette
50 calories, 5 g fat, 3 g carbs ✓

Renée's Wellness Dressing – pomegranate blueberry açai
30 calories, 0 g fat, 6 g carbs ✓

Toasted sliced almonds
100 calories, 8.5 g fat, 3.5 g carbs ✓

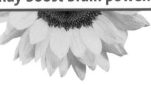

Studies show sunflower seeds may boost brain power.

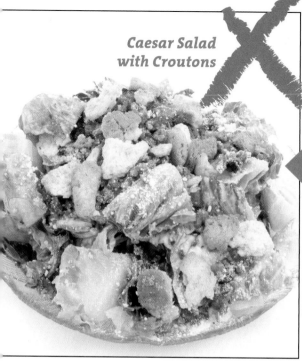

Caesar Salad with Croutons

Nutritional Value	
SERVING	1 salad
CALORIES	700
FAT	62 g
CARBS	26 g
FIBER	4 g
SUGAR	0 g
SODIUM	1,100 mg
PROTEIN	12 g

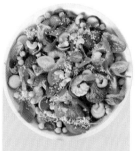

Ditch These Too!

Green Goddess dressing (2 oz)
260 calories, 24 g fat, 4 g carbs

Creamy Caesar dressing (2 oz)
190 calories, 18 g fat, 4 g carbs

Thousand Island dressing (2 oz)
210 calories, 19.9 g fat, 9.1 g carbs

▶ Nix "crispy" options such as fried chicken, croutons and noodles.

▶ Use only half the packet of dressing. The average packet contains two fluid ounces (four tablespoons!) and can pack on over 200 calories.

▶ Avoid salads with names such as "Caesar," "Taco" or "Southwestern."

▶ Pick a salad with fresh fruits and unsalted nuts.

SALAD SAVVY ▶ ▶ ▶ ▶ ▶ ▶ ▶

Fast-food salads make great on-the-run lunches. But if you've ever doubted the nutritional value of pairing a taco and salad, you're more salad savvy than you might think. A serving of Taco Bell's Fresco Style Fiesta taco salad has 750 calories and 37 grams of fat – equivalent to a Taco Supreme and a side of fries! Next time you're up at the counter, follow these tips:

Navigate your way around any salad bar — the fit way — and come out with a low-fat muscle-building meal. Then take your salad smarts home and try one of *Oxygen*'s two-minute dressings.

BY JULIE UPTON, MS, RD

IS YOUR SALAD MAKING YOU **FAT?**

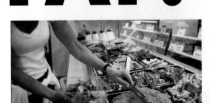

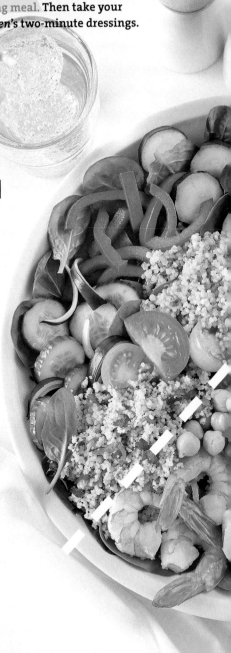

You may know your way around the weight room, but how about around the salad bar? If your leafy greens are buried under a heap of dressing, cheese, croutons and other toppings, you can wind up with a salad that has more calories and fat than a fast-food burger. The key to a better salad is to use a variety of nutrient-rich and low-calorie ingredients, and set portion limits on the number of toppings.

Now here's what you should scoop up, how much, and why your body will thank you.

 50% VEGGIES AND GRAINS

START: Pile on two to three vegetable servings. A serving counts as one cup of leafy greens or half a cup of any steamed vegetables. They're considered freebies because they're low in calories but deliver mighty vitamins beneficial to your fat-loss and muscle-building goals. **CHOOSE:** Spinach, kale, romaine, arugula, broccoli, peppers, tomatoes, cauliflower, onions, mushrooms, squash, cucumbers and all plain vegetables. **WHY:** Evidence shows that active women need more B vitamins, such as folic acid, for cell repair. Weightlifting causes micro tears in your muscles, making them vulnerable to free-radical damage (cell destruction). The antioxidants in vegetables help muscles recover after workouts. Fiber helps with weight management by increasing satiety so you'll feel fuller on fewer calories. **GO GREENER:** One cup of romaine lettuce gets you three times more folic acid than a cup of iceberg. Spinach and kale contain plentiful amounts of lipoic acid, an antioxidant proven to stifle the hunger pang hormone ghrelin and increase the "I'm full" hormone leptin. It has also been shown to help increase energy.

ADD: A half-cup of whole grains.
WHY: Complex carbohydrates will deliver a steady surge of energy by releasing insulin at a slower pace, keeping you fuller longer – without added fat.
CHOOSE: Cooked bulgur, couscous or protein-packed quinoa.

 25% HEALTHY FATS

STAY FULL: Add monounsaturated fat.
CHOOSE: One tablespoon of low-fat dressing plus one ounce of aged cheese or avocado (visualize two dice); or one-quarter cup of unsalted nuts.
WHY: Your body actually needs a bit of fat to absorb key nutrients from the vegetables, such as vitamin E, an antioxidant that helps in post-exercise muscle repair. **BEST CHEESE:** Count on lots of flavor with feta, blue or aged Parmesan, and you'll end up saving calories because you'll use less.

 25% LEAN PROTEIN

MUSCLE UP: Put three ounces of lean protein on top of your veggies and grains. **CHOOSE:** Eggs, tuna (without mayo), grilled fish, shrimp, lean turkey breast, skinless chicken breast, tofu, seeds or beans. **WHY:** By pairing up proper portions of complex carbs (vegetables and grains) and protein, you're optimizing your glycogen stores (energy source) making it possible for you to work out longer and lift heavier.
BEST VEG OPTION: Black beans are one of the best sources of protein and fiber a vegetarian can choose, and you'll get more antioxidants per serving than virtually anything else at the salad bar.

TWO MINUTES TO YOUR
BEST **HOMEMADE DRESSING**

Now that you have the ideal ingredients and portions down pat, you can start creating perfect salads at home without doubt. Instead of using that lone balsamic vinaigrette spritzer in your fridge again, whip up your own low-fat dressing. BY JULIE UPTON, MS, RD

Instructions for all dressings: *Whisk all ingredients in a bowl. Serve immediately or pour and seal in a bottle/jar. Refrigerate for up to seven days.*

SENSORY OVERLOAD!

When faced with a hundred different ingredients (like at the salad bar at Whole Foods), the temptation to pile on more than you need is inevitable. Research shows that when you are given a wider variety of foods to eat, you eat more. Consider the last time you dropped more than just a dollop of mayo-laden potato salad atop your already dressed greens – just to get a little taste of everything. Or when you tossed in a fistful of croutons, assuming they're just miniature toasts, not realizing manufacturers drizzle butter on them so they stay crunchy. Before you knew it, you were eating a 700-calorie fat trap. The scientific term used to describe this phenomenon is sensory-specific satiety. The more tastes and textures available to us, the more we'll eat – simple science.

ORANGE POPPY SEED DRESSING

Makes 6 servings

½ cup nonfat plain yogurt

¼ cup orange juice concentrate, thawed

2 Tbsp poppy seeds

1 Tbsp honey (optional)

Nutrients per serving: Calories: 60, Total Fats: 2 g, Saturated Fat: 0 g, Trans Fat: 0 g, Cholesterol: 0 mg, Sodium: 10 mg, Total Carbohydrates: 10 g, Dietary Fiber: 0 g, Sugar: 8 g, Protein: 2 g, Iron: 0.5 mg

SOY GINGER SESAME DRESSING

Makes 6 servings

½ cup nonfat sour cream

1 ½ Tbsp light soy sauce

3 Tbsp rice wine vinegar

2 tsp minced garlic

1 Tbsp Stevia

1 Tbsp sesame seeds

Nutrients per serving: Calories: 50, Total Fats: 2 g, Saturated Fat: 0 g, Trans Fat: 0 g, Cholesterol: 5 mg, Sodium: 250 mg, Total Carbohydrates: 8 g, Dietary Fiber: 0 g, Sugar: 4 g, Protein: 2 g, Iron: <0.5 mg

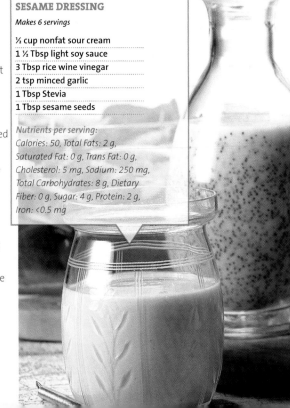

FLAXSEED OIL DRESSING

Makes 12 servings

¾ cup flaxseed oil

¼ cup red wine vinegar

½ tsp Dijon mustard

½ tsp maple syrup

½ tsp crushed garlic

½ tsp oregano

Nutrients per serving:
Calories: 80, Total Fats: 9 g,
Saturated Fat: 1 g, Trans Fat: 0 g,
Cholesterol: 0 mg, Sodium:
5 mg, Total Carbohydrates: 0 g,
Dietary Fiber: 0 g, Sugar: 0 g,
Protein: 0 g, Iron: 0 mg

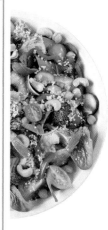

TIP
Another option for a quick, low-fat dressing is to use olive oil and vinegar but instead of mixing half of each, use a two to one ratio of vinegar to olive oil.

AVOCADO OIL & VINEGAR DRESSING

Makes 6 servings

¼ cup avocado oil

1 Tbsp rice vinegar

1 Tbsp honey

Juice of 1 lemon

¼ tsp sea salt

Nutrients per serving:
Calories: 100, Total Fats: 9 g, Saturated Fat: 1 g, Trans Fat: 0 g, Cholesterol: 0 mg, Sodium: 80 mg, Total Carbohydrates: 4 g, Dietary Fiber: 0 g, Sugar: 3 g, Protein: 0 g, Iron: 1 mg

HONEY DIJON DRESSING

Makes 6 servings

1 cup nonfat plain yogurt

1 ½ Tbsp Dijon mustard

2 Tbsp honey

1 tsp balsamic vinegar

Ground pepper, to taste

Nutrients per serving:
Calories: 40, Total Fats: 0 g,
Saturated Fat: 0 g, Trans Fat: 0 g,
Cholesterol: 0 mg, Sodium:
115 mg, Total Carbohydrates:
10 g, Dietary Fiber: 0 g,
Sugar: 8 g, Protein: 2 g, Iron: 0 mg

PICK IT

Nutritional Value	
SERVING	1 slice
CALORIES	240
FAT	9 g
CARBS	30 g
FIBER	2 g
SUGAR	6 g
SODIUM	710 mg
PROTEIN	10 g

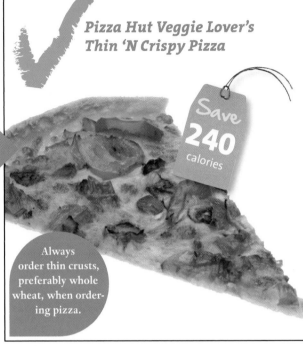

Pizza Hut Veggie Lover's Thin 'N Crispy Pizza

Save
240
calories

Always order thin crusts, preferably whole wheat, when ordering pizza.

MAKE IT BETTER

Order the green pepper, red onion and diced red tomato Fit 'n Delicious pizza for only 150 calories and 400 mg sodium per slice.

TIP Eat a salad first – you'll get extra nutrients and the salad will fill you up, making you less likely to overeat. Make sure to order dressing on the side!

Give It a Try!

Amy's frozen pizza – mushroom and olive
250 calories, 9 g fat, 33 g carbs

Whole Foods 365 Mediterranean pizza
180 calories, 8 g fat, 21 g carbs

Kashi Mediterranean pizza
290 calories, 9 g fat, 37 g carbs

Say What?

EATING A SLICE of cheese- and meat-loaded pizza can actually make you crave more foods that are high in saturated fat (butter, cheese, milk and beef) for up to three days, according to a study from UT Southwestern Medical Center. Researchers say eating a high-fat food, even once, "hits" your brain with fatty acids and prevents the hunger-regulating hormones – leptin and insulin – from signaling you to stop eating.

KICK IT

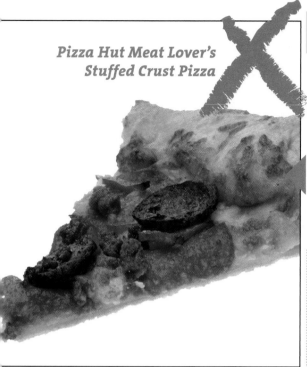

Pizza Hut Meat Lover's Stuffed Crust Pizza

Nutritional Value	
SERVING	1 slice
CALORIES	480
FAT	26 g
CARBS	39 g
FIBER	2 g
SUGAR	5 g
SODIUM	1,370 mg
PROTEIN	22 g

EAT WITH A MAN TO LOSE WEIGHT?

You may eat less if your lunch mate is a man, not a woman, according to the latest research. As reported in the online version of *Appetite*, your choice of food for lunch or dinner is often influenced by who is sitting across from you. As determined in a study from McMaster University, women who ate with a male companion ate significantly fewer calories than if they ate with a female. In addition, the more men in the group, the less the women ate. More men = fewer calories. Study author Meredith Young speculated that when women choose smaller, healthier portions, they appear more attractive to men.

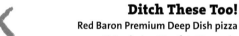

Ditch These Too!

Red Baron Premium Deep Dish pizza
420 calories, 19 g fat, 45 g carbs

Tony's Pizza Supreme – sausage & pepperoni
420 calories, 20 g fat, 43 g carbs

Garlic bread
170 calories, 7 g fat, 24 g carbs

>> FAST FACT

Whole wheat dough contains thiamin, which helps convert glucose (blood sugar) into energy.

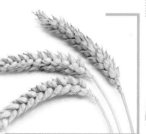

Try This

Blot the oil off the top of your pizza slice with paper towel — you'll save fat and calories!

PICK IT

Nutritional Value	
SERVING	2 Tbsp
CALORIES	35
FAT	3 g
CARBS	1 g
FIBER	0 g
SUGAR	1 g
SODIUM	75 mg
PROTEIN	1 g

Try This

Healthy dips can be used in wraps, on sandwiches, on baked potatoes or anywhere else you want a bit of pizzazz.

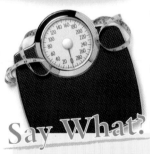

Light Cream Cheese Dip

Save **25** calories

Give It a Try!
Low-fat ricotta cheese with herbs
60 calories, 3 g fat, 3 g carbs

Guacamole
110 calories, 13 g fat, 5 g carbs

Tzatziki
30 calories, 2.5 g fat, 2 g carbs ✓

Say What?

NEED TO LOSE WEIGHT? LOOK BEYOND YOUR BMI.

A recent study published in *Nutrition Journal* demonstrated that looking at BMI alone led to fewer weight-loss recommendations, as compared with an analysis of waist circumference, percentage body fat and metabolic syndrome risk. Study authors have concluded that the consideration of BMI alone could lead to "unfortunate misclassifications" in identifying patients in need of lifestyle changes. Next time you step on the scale at your doctor's office, get all your questions answered.

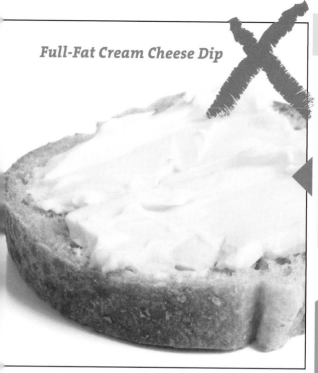

Full-Fat Cream Cheese Dip

Nutritional Value	
SERVING	2 Tbsp
CALORIES	60
FAT	4.5 g
CARBS	3 g
FIBER	0 g
SUGAR	0 g
SODIUM	200 mg
PROTEIN	1 g

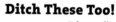

ALL YOU!

If you've ever wanted to own a dog, follow your instincts. According to the CDC, you can go a long way toward better health with a dog by your side. And recent research in *Obesity* found that people with pooches were also more likely to lose weight. A walk with your best pal after dinner can go a long way toward losing weight and staying on track.

Ditch These Too!

7-layer dip
250 calories, 14 g fat, 11.5 g carbs

Kraft Cheez Whiz
90 calories, 7 g fat, 4 g carbs

Stop & Shop veggie dip
120 calories, 12 g fat, 2 g carbs

YES YOU CAN

Get on the ball! **Stability balls are a great alternative to a chair at the office. Sitting on one at your desk can burn up to 85 calories every 30 minutes.**

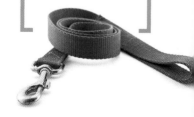

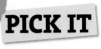

PICK IT

California Roll

Love This!

Nutritional Value	
SERVING	8 pieces (1 roll)
CALORIES	300
FAT	8 g
CARBS	50 g
FIBER	4 g
SUGAR	5 g
SODIUM	340 mg
PROTEIN	8 g

Save 240 calories

Give It A Try!

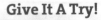

✅ **Edamame (soybeans)**
156 calories, 8 g fat, 12 g carbs

✅ **Sashimi (sliced raw seafood)**
122 calories, 1.1 g fat, 0 carbs

✅ **Brown rice salmon roll**
437 calories, 18 g fat, 46 g carbs

tip Eating too quickly not only messes with your digestion, it makes you eat more than you normally would. To slow down, try eating with chopsticks.

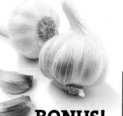

IF YOU SLOW DOWN AND EAT LESS, YOU WILL ENJOY YOUR FOOD MORE – A REVELATION FROM A RESEARCH STUDY AT THE UNIVERSITY OF RHODE ISLAND.

KICK IT

Tempura Roll

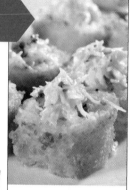

AVOID FOODS THAT SAY "TEMPURA" AT THE SUSHI BAR. THIS IS A CODE WORD FOR "DEEP FRIED."

BONUS!

Flavorful ingredients such as pepper, ginger, garlic and cumin can heat up your meal – and your fat burning! A study out of the Netherlands concluded that these ingredients have a significant effect on thermogenesis, which raises your metabolism. Make sure to munch some pickled ginger and wasabi with your sushi.

76

Percentage of adults that say they are trying to eat more healthfully now at restaurants than they did two years ago.

– NATIONAL RESTAURANT ASSOCIATION, 2009 RESAURANT INDUSTRY FORECAST

Go green. Studies show that green tea burns fat! Switch your sugar- and dairy-doused coffee for a green tea bag a few times a week.

YES YOU CAN

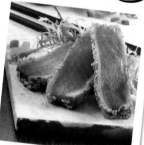

Nutritional Value

SERVING	8 pieces (1 roll)
CALORIES	540
FAT	12 g
CARBS	82 g
FIBER	4 g
SUGAR	15 g
SODIUM	1,120 mg
PROTEIN	26 g

Ditch These Too!

Beef teriyaki
249 calories, 14.5 g fat, 2.5 g carbs

Sake (wine)
155 calories, 0 fat, 5.8 g carbs

Cream cheese with crab roll
440 calories, 14 g fat, 66.8 g carbs

SAY WHAT? You get a wide choice at today's sushi restaurants. Omega-3-rich fish such as salmon, tuna and mackerel are great nutrient-rich sushi options (don't forget that yellowfin or ahi tuna contains less mercury than albacore tuna). NOTE: If you're pregnant, you may not want to take the risk of eating raw fish sushi at all – talk to your doctor, first.

PICK IT

McDonald's Chipotle BBQ Snack Wrap (Grilled), Small Fries, 1% Milk

Nutritional Value	
SERVING	1 of each item
CALORIES	600
FAT	22 g
CARBS	69 g
FIBER	4 g
SUGAR	17 g
SODIUM	1,110 mg
PROTEIN	29 g

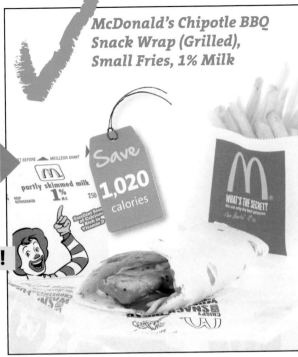

Save **1,020** calories

BONUS!

More Americans are paying attention to prices and some are switching to cheaper restaurants. Many customers are cutting out booze, desserts and appetizers to make their meals less expensive. Restaurants, realizing that Americans are worried about the economy but still want to eat out, are offering "recession deals" – prix fixe three-course lunches or dinners or bistro-styled cost-cutting dinners. There are Frugal Fridays, two-for-one sushi specials and half-price appetizers.

– National Restaurant Association

Give It a Try!

McDonald's Snack Size Fruit & Walnut Salad
210 calories, 8 g fat, 31 g carbs

McDonald's Honey Mustard Chicken Snack Wrap (grilled)
240 calories, 9 g fat, 24 g carbs

McDonald's Latte with nonfat milk
90 calories, 0 fat, 13 g carbs

Say What?

CALCIUM has been proven to rev up your fat-burning potential. Get your fix from low-fat dairy, soy products and dark green veggies. Also, calcium gives bones both strength and rigidity, especially as you age.

McDonald's Chicken Selects (5 pcs), Medium Fries and Chocolate Shake (16 oz)

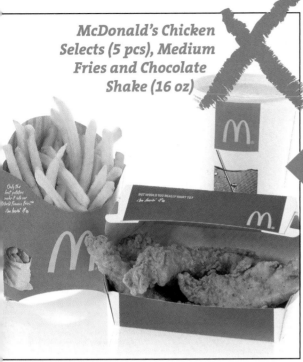

KICK IT

Nutritional Value	
SERVING	1 of each item
CALORIES	1,620
FAT	72 g
CARBS	188 g
FIBER	6 g
SUGAR	84 g
SODIUM	2,200 mg
PROTEIN	55 g

TIP Don't eat lunch at your desk. Studies show that grazing while gazing at a computer screen leads to indiscriminate calorie consumption.

91

Percentage of women who admit to having food cravings. Researchers found that people continue to experience cravings even six months into a diet. The study suggests giving in to cravings once in a while for successful weight loss (but don't take this as permission to binge!).

-Tufts University

Ditch These Too!

McDonald's Double Quarter Pounder with Cheese
740 calories, 42 g fat, 40 g carbs

McDonald's Crispy Chicken Ranch BLT
580 calories, 23 g fat, 61 g carbs

McDonald's McFlurry (12 fl oz)
550 calories, 17 g fat, 88 g carbs

» FAST FACT

Magnesium aids in the absorption of calcium, helps maintain heart health and blood pressure levels, and promotes muscle function. Magnesium maximizes your energy and staves off annoying muscular cramps. Get yours from almonds, halibut and bran cereals.

PICK IT

Nutritional Value	
SERVING	1
CALORIES	319
FAT	4.5 g
CARBS	48.4 g
FIBER	5.5 g
SUGAR	7 g
SODIUM	743 mg
PROTEIN	23 g

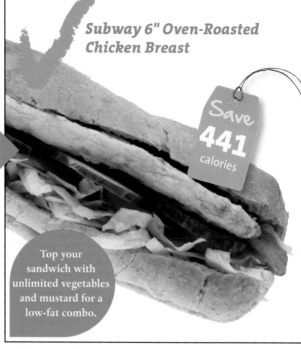

Subway 6" Oven-Roasted Chicken Breast

Save **441** calories

Top your sandwich with unlimited vegetables and mustard for a low-fat combo.

MAKE IT BETTER

Order the 9-grain wheat bread for double the fiber of Italian bread.

EVEN BETTER

Have the Subway employee scoop out the inside of the bun for fewer calories and starchy carbs.

Give It a Try!

Turkey Breast Mini Sub (9-grain wheat bread)
279 calories, 14 g fat, 26 g carbs

6" Veggie Delite (six grams of fat or less)
229 calories, 2.2 g fat, 44.9 g carbs

Oven Roasted Chicken Salad (with fat-free Italian dressing)
160 calories, 2.5 g fat, 16 g carbs

YES YOU CAN

Practice deep cleansing breaths to curb cortisol spikes that can sabotage your fat-loss program. Learn a deep-breathing exercise and do it at least once a day to help control your stress levels and avoid chronic cortisol release. Remember this mantra: "Chronic cortisol leads to bigger guts and larger butts; breathing well cuts the swell."

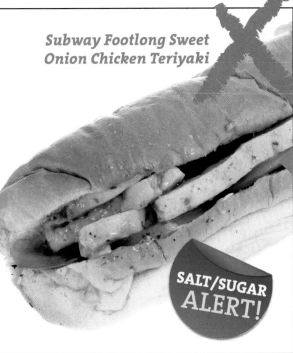

Subway Footlong Sweet Onion Chicken Teriyaki

SALT/SUGAR ALERT!

KICK IT

Nutritional Value	
SERVING	1
CALORIES	760
FAT	9 g
CARBS	120 g
FIBER	10 g
SUGAR	34 g
SODIUM	2,020 mg
PROTEIN	51 g

Say What?

AMERICANS NOW spend almost 50 percent of their food dollars away from home – the highest percentage on record. Only 37 percent of those food dollars were spent away from home 30 years ago, and 50 years ago, that figure was just 25 percent.

– U.S. Department of Agriculture's Economic Research Service

Ditch These Too!

6" Meatball Marinara
580 calories, 23 g fat, 70 g carbs, 1,530 mg sodium

6" Feast (turkey, black forest ham, roast beef, genoa salami, pepperoni, cheese, veggies)
540 calories, 22 g fat, 50 g carbs, 2,470 mg sodium

Footlong Subway Club
640 calories, 10 g fat, 95 g carbs

>> **FAST FACT**

New York City is taking aim at the amount of salt in packaged foods. In fact, it's the first city to implement the National Salt Reduction Initiative's move to cut "hidden" salt by 25 percent over the next five years. The group has goals to help companies reduce sodium in 61 categories of packaged foods, plus 25 types of restaurants. Flip to chapter seven to find out more about sodium levels in your food.

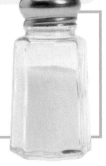

SANDWICHES: Try These

ROAST BEEF ON SOURDOUGH

Ready in 5 minutes • Makes 1 serving

½ Tbsp plain low-fat yogurt

1 oz blue (Stilton) cheese, crumbled

2 slices sourdough bread

4 oz lean roast beef, thinly sliced

¼ cup spinach

⅛ red onion, thinly sliced

Mix together yogurt and cheese. Spread on one slice of sourdough bread. Top with roast beef, spinach, onion and remaining slice of bread.

Nutrients per serving:
Calories: 477, Total Fats: 21 g, Saturated Fat: 5 g, Trans Fat: 0 g, Cholesterol: 92 mg, Sodium: 472 mg, Total Carbohydrates: 35 g, Dietary Fiber: <0.5 g, Sugar: 2 g, Protein: 37 g, Iron: 2 mg

CARBS YOU MUST EAT

It's no surprise that you should stay away from white bread. Not only does it lead it to energy slumps, but white refined bread also falls short on nutrients that help with fat and muscle metabolism. But if you still crave the taste of white bread, **eat sourdough.** Like white bread, sourdough contains processed and bleached white flour, but it also contains lactic acid (produced after processing to give it that sour taste), which breaks down the sugar content. As a result, sourdough is a low-glycemic carbohydrate that keeps insulin levels low and provides enough carbs for muscle growth.

EZEKIEL BREAD is a great carbohydrate choice for boosting lean muscle gains because of its complete protein profile. Ezekiel is made from legumes and soybeans. Soy protein, in particular, contains high amounts of arginine and glutamine, two amino acids that help promote muscle growth. This Caesar sandwich is a far cry from a standard high-fat Caesar salad, which can fatten you up with up to 700 calories and 50 grams of fat! Stay in fat-fighting shape with our sandwich version instead.

TURKEY CAESAR ON EZEKIEL

Ready in 5 minutes • Makes 1 serving

½ Tbsp Parmesan cheese, grated

1 Tbsp low-fat mayonnaise

1 tsp lemon juice

1 dash Worcestershire sauce

Sea salt and pepper, to taste

2 slices Ezekiel bread, toasted

4 oz roasted turkey breast, thinly sliced

1 romaine lettuce leaf

Mix together cheese, mayonnaise, lemon juice, Worcestershire sauce, salt and pepper. Spread on one slice of toast. Top with turkey, lettuce and remaining slice of toast.

Nutrients per serving:
Calories: 344, Total Fats: 4 g, Saturated Fat: 1 g, Trans Fat: 0 g, Cholesterol: 3 mg, Sodium: 361 mg, Total Carbohydrates: 32 g, Dietary Fiber: 6 g, Sugar: 0 g, Protein: 45 g, Iron: 3 mg

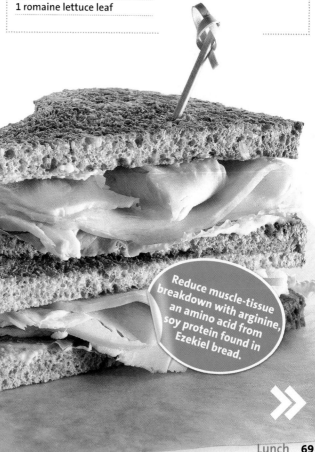

Reduce muscle-tissue breakdown with arginine, an amino acid from soy protein found in Ezekiel bread.

BBQ CHICKEN PITA POCKET

Ready in 5 minutes • Makes 1 serving

- 1 skinless chicken breast, grilled on the barbeque
- 1 Tbsp low-sugar barbeque sauce
- 1 whole wheat pita pocket, cut in half
- ¼ cup romaine lettuce, thinly sliced
- ¼ avocado, sliced
- 1 Tbsp corn kernels
- 1 oz low-fat cheddar cheese

Shred chicken and toss with barbeque sauce. Open pita pocket halves and place lettuce at the bottom. Layer chicken, avocado, corn and cheese.

Nutrients per serving:
Calories: 382, Total Fats: 10 g, Saturated Fat: 3 g, Trans Fat: 0 g, Cholesterol: 79 mg, Sodium: 636 mg, Total Carbohydrates: 34 g, Dietary Fiber: 5 g, Sugar: 1 g, Protein: 39 g, Iron: 2 mg

Crush 3:00 p.m. snack cravings by adding a healthy fat into your lunch. Try a slice of avocado, a source of monounsaturated fats.

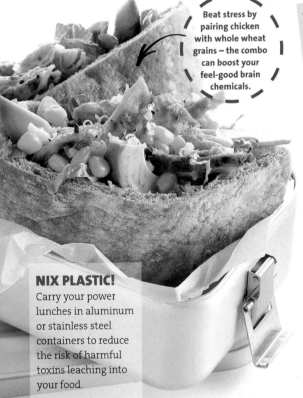

Beat stress by pairing chicken with whole wheat grains – the combo can boost your feel-good brain chemicals.

TIME-SAVING TIP
Replace barbequed chicken with a can of chicken breast, drained.

CARBS YOU MUST EAT

WHOLE WHEAT PITA

pockets are surprisingly very low in sugar. One large pocket can have less than a gram of sugar whereas two slices of whole wheat bread boasts about six grams. Less sugar means no mid-afternoon crash and burn. Whole wheat varieties are also packed with B vitamins, specifically vitamin B-6, which can help fight fatigue. Stuff your pocket with chicken and you may feel more motivated to hit the gym, even after a stressful day at work. Chicken and whole wheat breads contain tryptophan, an amino acid that can lower your stress levels.

NIX PLASTIC!
Carry your power lunches in aluminum or stainless steel containers to reduce the risk of harmful toxins leaching into your food.

SALMON BLT ON RYE

Ready in 5 minutes • Makes 1 serving

- **2 slices rye bread**
- **1 Tbsp low-fat herbed cream cheese**
- **3 oz salmon filet, grilled or baked**
- **2 pieces turkey bacon, cooked**
- **1 slice tomato**
- **1 leaf Boston lettuce**

Toast both pieces of rye bread. Spread cream cheese over one piece of toast. Layer with salmon, turkey bacon, tomato and lettuce. Top with remaining slice of toast.

Nutrients per serving:
Calories: 355, Total Fats: 11 g, Saturated Fat: 2.1 g, Trans Fat: 0 g, Cholesterol: 77 mg, Sodium: 650 mg, Total Carbohydrates: 31 g, Dietary Fiber: 3 g, Sugar: 1 g, Protein: 33 g, Iron: 2.7 mg

EAT SALMON twice a week to help lower triglycerides, a form of fat left in your bloodstream from consuming more calories than your body needs.

CARBS YOU MUST EAT

RYE BREAD kernels have been shown to slow digestion, which will help keep you full and energized by keeping your blood-sugar levels steady all afternoon. Like whole wheat, rye is high in energy-boosting manganese and muscle-building protein. If you're trying to build muscle without gaining excess fat, rye can help because it is especially rich with noncellulose polysaccharides, a type of fiber that can quickly give you a feeling of fullness. But be cautious when choosing rye. If the first listed ingredient is "unbleached enriched flour" you won't get as much fiber. Muscle-up rye bread's rich, hearty taste with low-fat turkey bacon and salmon.

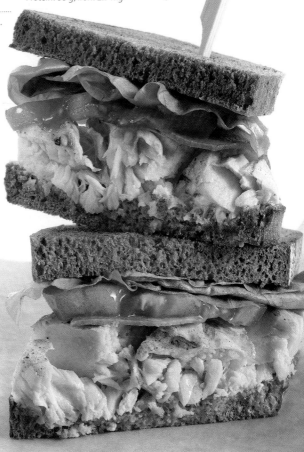

PICK IT

Nutritional Value

SERVING	1 taco
CALORIES	170
FAT	4 g
CARBS	21 g
FIBER	3 g
SUGAR	3 g
SODIUM	730 mg
PROTEIN	12 g

Taco Bell Ranchero Chicken Soft Taco (Fresco Style)

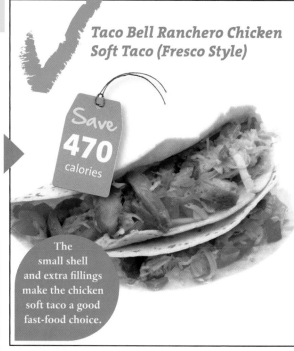

Save **470** calories

The small shell and extra fillings make the chicken soft taco a good fast-food choice.

MAKE IT BETTER

Order "Fresco Style" to save even more calories.

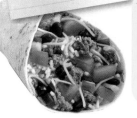

REALLY HUNGRY? Double up on the tacos and still eat fewer calories than in one burrito.

Give It a Try!

Taco Salad (without shell)
460 calories, 23 g fat, 41 g carbs ✓

Grilled steak soft taco (Fresco style)
160 calories, 4.5 g fat, 20 g carbs ✓

Chicken quesadillas
520 calories, 28 g fat, 40 g carbs ✓

Say What?

DUTCH RESEARCHERS looked at more than 20,000 men and women in their 40s and determined that larger waist sizes were associated with higher rates of cardiovascular disease. In fact, over a 10-year period, women with waists greater than 34.5 inches were almost three times more likely to suffer from heart disease.

Taco Bell Grilled Stuffed Burrito with Chicken

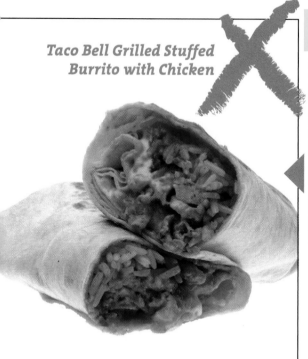

KICK IT

Nutritional Value	
SERVING	1 burrito
CALORIES	640
FAT	23 g
CARBS	73 g
FIBER	7 g
SUGAR	6 g
SODIUM	2,160 mg
PROTEIN	34 g

50

Percentage by which the American Public Health Association has called for a reduction of salt in restaurant and processed food over the next 10 years. This action may save 150,000 lives every year from strokes, heart disease and other illnesses exacerbated by excess sodium.
– University of Maryland Medical Center

Ditch These Too!

Fully loaded taco salads
200 calories, 12 g fat, 15 g carbs

Bell Grande nachos
760 calories, 42 g fat, 77 g carbs

Volcano burrito
800 calories, 42 g fat, 81 g carbs

YES YOU CAN

MAKE TACOS YOURSELF AND SAVE CALORIES AND FAT!
A family favorite that does double duty – you not only control portion size (one of the major factors in an unhealthy diet), you save money! Plus, your family will love the choices – simply buy a package of soft tacos (or hard ones for those picky family members), grate low-fat cheese, cut up tomatoes, green peppers and grilled chicken. Presto! Homemade tacos at a fraction of the cost and calories!

PICK IT

Nutritional Value	
SERVING	1 taco
CALORIES	330
FAT	7 g
CARBS	54 g
FIBER	9 g
SUGAR	4 g
SODIUM	1,200 mg
PROTEIN	12 g

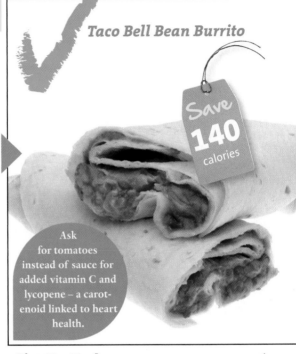

Taco Bell Bean Burrito

Save **140** calories

Ask for tomatoes instead of sauce for added vitamin C and lycopene – a carotenoid linked to heart health.

EXCUSE BUSTED

I'm too tired to work out.

Working out will improve your energy levels, so unless you're sick or didn't sleep the night before, get to the gym and those pumping endorphins will prove you wrong. In fact, there's no pick-me-up like a good workout!

TIP Pack black beans in your burrito instead of refried beans and save 250 calories a cup!

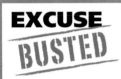

Give It a Try!
Salsa
20 calories, 0 fat, 4 g carbs

Mexican rice
110 calories, 3 g fat, 19 g carbs

Beef soft taco
200 calories, 9 g fat, 21 g carbs

BONUS!

Foods with lots
of fiber and protein help stabilize your blood sugar and keep you feeling full for hours, and beans are chock full of both!

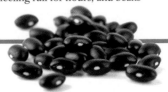

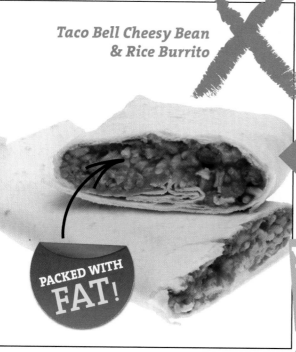

Taco Bell Cheesy Bean & Rice Burrito

KICK IT

Nutritional Value	
SERVING	1 taco
CALORIES	470
FAT	20 g
CARBS	58 g
FIBER	6 g
SUGAR	5 g
SODIUM	1,400 mg
PROTEIN	13 g

PACKED WITH FAT!

YES YOU CAN

Keep your metabolism peaked. Eat smaller clean meals every two to three hours to burn more fat, to prevent energy sags and to think more clearly and effectively all day.

Ditch These Too!

 Sour cream
51 calories, 5 g fat, 1 g carbs

Cheesy Fiesta potatoes
270 calories, 15 g fat, 30 g carbs

Cheesy double beef burrito
460 calories, 20 g fat, 52 g carbs

Say What?

ADD PROTEIN to every meal and snack: small portions of chicken, nuts, beans, tofu or cheese. Protein takes more energy to digest, so you'll burn calories while you process them. Try this: combine meat and vegetarian sources of protein for added nutritional punch — for example, chili made with lean turkey and beans.

133 million

Number of Americans who eat out each day.
– National Restaurant Association

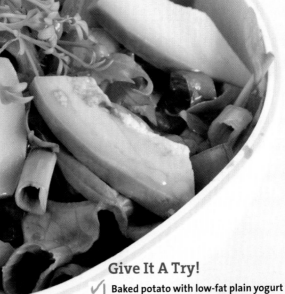

PICK IT

Avocado Salad

Love This!

Save **70** *calories*

Nutritional Value	
SERVING	¼ avocado
CALORIES	130
FAT	5 g
CARBS	21 g
FIBER	3 g
SUGAR	2 g
SODIUM	280 mg
PROTEIN	1 g

Give It A Try!

☑ **Baked potato with low-fat plain yogurt**
293 calories, 1 g fat, 65 g carbs

☑ **Baked potato with salsa and fresh cilantro**
287 calories, 0 fat, 65 g carbs

☑ **Mixed green salad with vinaigrette**
38 calories, 0 fat, 8 g carbs

GROWN IN
CALIFORNIA

AVOCADOS CONTAIN FOLATE, A B-VITAMIN CRUCIAL FOR WOMEN OF CHILD-BEARING AGE. IT HELPS ENSURE YOU HAVE A HEALTHY BABY.

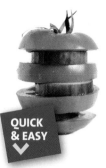

QUICK & EASY ▼

Eat fat to lose fat (really).
Eating enough "healthy" fats (but not too much) leaves you feeling more satisfied, so you're less likely to reach for extra food later on. Besides, you need fat for healthy skin, cells and even brain function. Just make sure you eat the right kinds.

YES YOU CAN

Mash a quarter of an avocado into one can of drained tuna. Add tomatoes, cucumbers and sea salt for flavor. Stuff inside a whole grain wrap for a satisfying lunch.

Choose California-grown avocados over Florida-grown. They have fewer calories and less sugar.

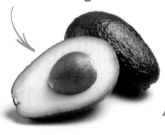

BONUS!

An avocado, rich in healthy monosaturated fat, has an added benefit – it has double the amount of potassium as a banana. (But it's also high in calories, so go easy!)

> **SAY WHAT?** The American Dietetic Association (ADA) recommends that 25 to 30 percent of your calories come from healthy fats. Add some form of healthy fats (that contain Omega-3, Omega-6 and Omega-9 fatty acids) into at least two or three meals each day. Almonds, walnuts, pumpkin seeds, flaxseed, fatty fish, olive oil and avocados are all great choices.

KICK IT ✗

Potato Salad

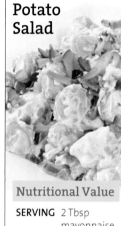

Nutritional Value

SERVING	2 Tbsp mayonnaise
CALORIES	200
FAT	10 g
CARBS	24 g
FIBER	3 g
SUGAR	5 g
SODIUM	540 mg
PROTEIN	2 g

Ditch These Too! ⟩

✗ **Baked potato with sour cream and chives**
320 calories, 3.5 g fat, 63 g carbs

✗ **Baked potato with cheese sauce and broccoli**
340 calories, 2.5 g fat, 70 g carbs

✗ **Creamy macaroni salad**
180 calories, 9 g fat, 20 g carbs

PICK IT

Nutritional Value

SERVING	3 slices
CALORIES	66
FAT	1.1 g
CARBS	2.6 g
FIBER	0.3 g
SUGAR	2.2 g
SODIUM	639 mg
PROTEIN	10.8 g

MAKE IT
BETTER

Forgo the deli and make your sandwich from sliced roasted chicken or turkey breast.

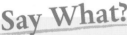

Turkey Breast Deli Meat

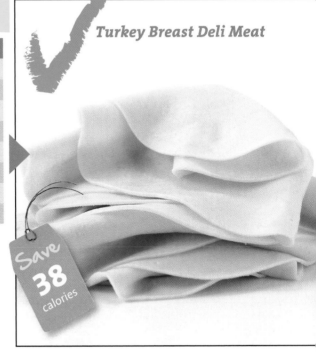

Save **38** calories

Give It a Try!

Fat-free bologna
25 calories, 0.5 g fat, 3 g carbs

Lean roast beef
70 calories, 1.5 g fat, 1 g carbs

Extra lean roasted ham
69 calories, 1.8 g fat, 1.6 g carbs

Say What?

BELIEVE IT OR NOT, the more you sleep, the slimmer you'll stay. "Getting enough sleep is essential to healthy eating habits," says Dr. Christine Gerbstadt, a dietician and spokesperson for the American Dietetic Association. "If you're getting fewer than seven hours of sleep, you're less likely to lose weight." Gerbstadt explains that lack of sleep raises levels of cortisol, a hormone that increases stress, blood pressure and blood sugar. Cortisol also inflates appetite, cravings for sugar and weight gain — so rest up to shape up!

Salami Deli Meat

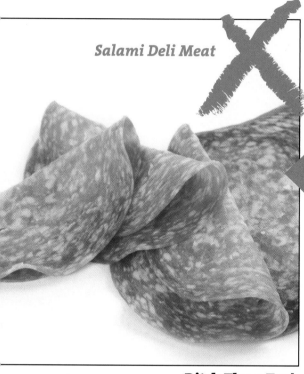

KICK IT

Nutritional Value	
SERVING	3 slices
CALORIES	104
FAT	8.1 g
CARBS	1 g
FIBER	0 g
SUGAR	0 g
SODIUM	543 mg
PROTEIN	6.3 g

> ## QUICK & EASY
Make a healthy sandwich by combining turkey breast meat, low-fat cheese, hummus, lettuce and tomatoes on whole wheat bread.

Ditch These Too!

Italian sausage
230 calories, 18.3 g fat, 2.9 g carbs

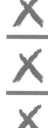

Spam with bacon
180 calories, 16 g fat, 1 g carbs

Pepperoni
135 calories, 11.7 g fat, 1.2 g carbs

Say What?

TODAY, in America, the most popular meal at lunch and dinner is a sandwich, with the top beverage listed as soda.

– The New York Times magazine, August 2, 2009 (data from the NPD Group)

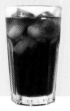

Pass on the mayonnaise **BONUS!**

for your sandwiches and use Dijon mustard instead – you'll not only enjoy the taste, you'll add a host of health benefits and eat fewer calories. Mustard seeds contain selenium and omega-3 fatty acids. They are also a good source of phosphorus, magnesium, manganese, dietary fiber, iron, calcium, protein, niacin and zinc.

PICK IT

Nutritional Value	
SERVING	1 Tbsp
CALORIES	23
FAT	1.3 g
CARBS	2 g
FIBER	0.8 g
SUGAR	0 g
SODIUM	53 mg
PROTEIN	1.1 g

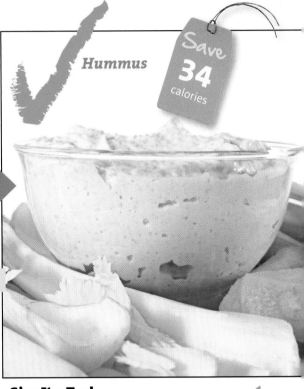

Hummus

Save 34 calories

BONUS!

Chickpeas
can be dried and used as flour in gluten-free recipes.

Try This

All you need is a blender! Purée garbanzo beans, olive oil, fresh garlic, tahini and lemon juice to make a quick and easy hummus spread.

Give It a Try!

Tzatziki (1 Tbsp)
15 calories, 1.3 g fat, 1 g carbs

Baba ghannouj (1 Tbsp)
55 calories, 6 g fat, 0.5 g carbs

Bruschetta (2 Tbsp)
30 calories, 2.5 g fat, 2 g carbs

Say What?

CHICKPEAS, like many other beans, are a good source of cholesterol-lowering fiber. And that provides an extra bonus – it prevents blood sugar levels from rising too rapidly after a meal, making these beans an especially good choice for individuals with diabetes, insulin resistance or hypoglycemia. Add them to whole grains such as rice or a whole wheat pita, and you've got a great high-quality protein.

Mayonnaise

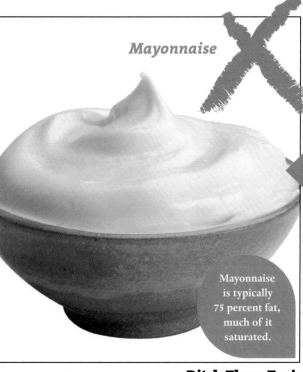

> Mayonnaise is typically 75 percent fat, much of it saturated.

KICK IT

Nutritional Value

SERVING	1 Tbsp
CALORIES	57
FAT	4.9 g
CARBS	3.5 g
FIBER	0 g
SUGAR	0.9 g
SODIUM	105 mg
PROTEIN	0.1 g

❯ QUICK & EASY

- Chunks of cauliflower
- Slices of green and red peppers
- Baby carrots
- Hummus for dipping

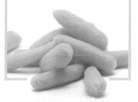

Ditch These Too!

Kraft Cheez Whiz (1 Tbsp)
45 calories, 3.5 g fat, 2 g carbs

Stop & Shop veggie dip
120 calories, 12 g fat, 2 g carbs

Snacks To Go bagel and cream cheese
240 calories, 9 g fat, 34 g carbs

PLUS!

Eating high-fiber foods helps prevent heart disease, according to findings in the *Archives of Internal Medicine*.

FAST FACT »

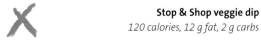

Chickpeas are one of the oldest known cultivated legumes and have been found in archeological digs throughout the Middle East at sites up to 12,000 years old.

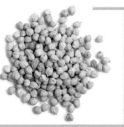

PICK IT

Nutritional Value	
SERVING	4 oz
CALORIES	131
FAT	0.9 g
CARBS	0 g
FIBER	0 g
SUGAR	0 g
SODIUM	383 mg
PROTEIN	28.8 g

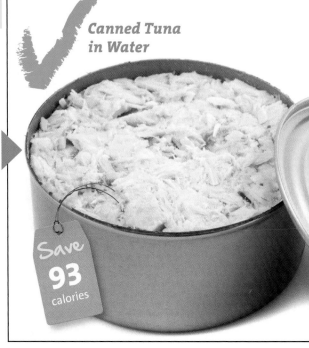

Canned Tuna in Water

Save
93
calories

MAKE IT BETTER

Drizzle tuna with lemon and grind some fresh pepper on top for a flavor boost.

Try This

Sip flavored sparkling water with lemon instead of soda, sweetened tea or lemonade.

Give It a Try!

Low-sodium canned tuna in water (4 oz)
120 calories, 1 g fat, 26 g carbs

Tuna chunk (in pouch) (4 oz)
180 calories, 2 g fat, 0 carbs

Salmon chunks in water (4 oz)
120 calories, 4 g fat, 0 carbs

FATTER, NOT FITTER

Canned chicken is higher in fat and calories because it often contains dark meat — not just lean breast meat.

▶ QUICK & EASY

Unzip a pouch of tuna packed in water for a low-cal protein boost.

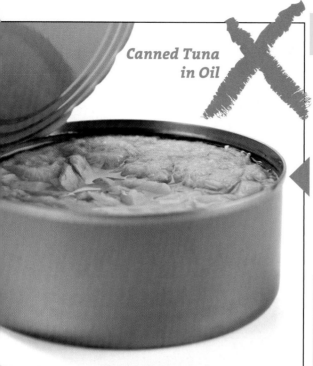

Canned Tuna in Oil

KICK IT

Nutritional Value	
SERVING	4 oz
CALORIES	224
FAT	9.3 g
CARBS	0 g
FIBER	0 g
SUGAR	0 g
SODIUM	400 mg
PROTEIN	32.9 g

Choose low-sodium tuna packed in water rather than oil and save five grams of fat per four ounces.

Ditch These Too!

Chicken roll (4 oz)
176 calories, 8.4 g fat, 2.7 g carbs

Canned full-fat corned beef
240 calories, 14 g fat, 0 carbs

Bumble Bee Lunch on the Run (tuna kit)
400 calories, 23.5 g fat, 38 g carbs

 FAST FACT
Albacore has a high mercury content. Choose chunk light tuna instead.

 YES YOU CAN
Eat healthfully at work. Keep a stock of tuna in cans or pouches and some unsalted nuts in your desk drawer to add to a garden salad. Try making your own healthy dressings — it's as easy as mixing some olive oil and flavored vinegar in a spritzer bottle, or just adding a squeeze of lemon.

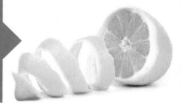

PICK IT

Nutritional Value	
SERVING	1 slice
CALORIES	65
FAT	1 g
CARBS	12.1 g
FIBER	1.7 g
SUGAR	2.6 g
SODIUM	127 mg
PROTEIN	2.6 g

TIP Those marketing devils are at it again. The word "multigrain" makes you think you're getting unprocessed grains, but if the first word you read is "enriched," those grains have been refined. And now that they know we've figured this out, they're up to their tricks again. If the ingredient list says "wheat flour," your brain says "whole wheat flour," but that's not the case unless it says so. Look for the word "whole" to ensure that the nutrient-rich germ and bran are intact.

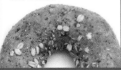

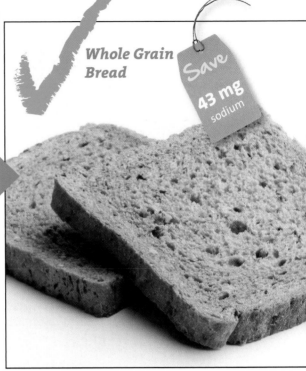

Whole Grain Bread

Save **43 mg** sodium

Give It a Try!

Rice cakes (1 cake)
35 calories, 0 fat, 7 g carbs

Mini whole grain pitas
65 calories, 0 fat, 14 g carbs

Trans-fat-free whole grain crackers
45 calories, 0.5 g fat, 9 g carbs

10,000

The number of steps you should be taking daily.

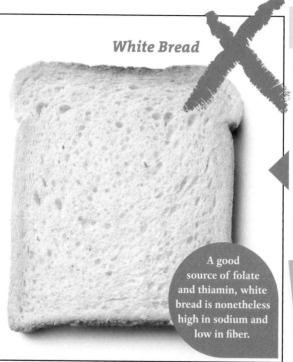

White Bread

A good source of folate and thiamin, white bread is nonetheless high in sodium and low in fiber.

KICK IT

Nutritional Value	
SERVING	1 slice
CALORIES	67
FAT	0.8 g
CARBS	12.7 g
FIBER	0.6 g
SUGAR	1.1 g
SODIUM	170 mg
PROTEIN	1.9 g

Try This

Eat starchy carbs early in the day and taper off at night. You'll burn them off during the day – they'll burn you at night. The only exception is after a long evening workout, when you do need carbs to replenish your energy.

Ditch These Too!

 Thickly sliced white bread
165 calories, 1.7 g fat, 31.7 g carbs

 Cornbread
200 calories, 7.5 g fat, 28 g carbs

 White hamburger buns
200 calories, 3 g fat, 37 g carbs

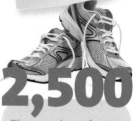

YES YOU CAN

Eat more to lose more. Just be smart about it. Choosing nutritious, clean food means you can eat more food, eat more often, stay satisfied and stay lean. What's not to like?

2,500

The number of *extra* steps a person takes when tracking steps on a pedometer. That's over a mile!
– *University of Michigan Health System*

SOUP'S ON!

Want a fat-loss secret? **A hearty bowl of slimming soup! Research shows that consuming soup helps you cut down on the overall calories in your meal by as much as 20 percent.** Slurp up!

PICK IT

Chicken & White Bean Soup

Celery is a low-cal (just 19 calories a cup!), high-fiber vegetable that provides a surprising number of nutrients — it may help reduce blood pressure and boost immunity. It's also a good source of potassium, folate and vitamin B6.

Protein-Packed!

Celery has the best flavor when it isn't overcooked — overcooking this vegetable can decrease its nutritional value by as much as half.

Add even more protein by adding grilled chicken breast, cut into one-inch chunks.

Celery is in season during the summer months. Although it's available year round, you'll enjoy the quality and taste more in the summer. Look for locally grown celery at farmers' markets for the best flavor.

Milder than onions or garlic, leeks boast many health benefits and nutrients — a good source of manganese, folate and Vitamin C. In addition, they also may contain similar heart-protecting qualities to those found in onions and garlic.

KICK IT
Cream of Broccoli Soup

Fat alert! Avoid cream-based soups – they can add as much as 100 more calories!

TOP TIP
Choose low-sodium chicken broth as the base for your soup.

Add beans to your diet and look forward to a magic food – nutrient-rich and protein-packed, they are inexpensive and versatile. Loaded with fiber, they are a great way to maintain a healthy weight.

5 Number of servings of beans and legumes you should be eating every week. Toss them into soups or salads and presto! They make a complete and hearty meal.

Spinach is low in calories (41 calories per cup), and loaded with iron, fiber, calcium, potassium and manganese. It's also high in vitamin K, which is important for blood and bone health. Bonus! It's fat-free.

In addition to its high nutrient value, particularly in heart-happy vitamins and minerals, spinach is good for your brain, vision and, of course, your muscles!

For more soups see next page

I love to sit down to a comforting bowl of soup, but this food can be a cunning culprit. Often deceptively high in sodium or fat, an innocent-looking bowl can be a diet downfall.

And yet research has proven that soups can be a great start to your meal. In fact, studies have shown that sipping soup can help you cut down on the overall calories of the rest of your meal by 20 percent, while helping you feel full for longer. Nutritionists suggest maximizing the nutrients and cutting the sodium in every bowl to maximize fat loss. Low-sodium, low-fat, broth-based soups are your best bet.

PICK IT

Love This!

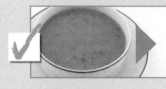

Lentil Soup

SERVING: 1 cup
CALORIES: 150
FAT: 2 g
CARBS: 28 g
FIBER: 5 g
SUGAR: 1 g
SODIUM: 870 mg
PROTEIN: 9 g

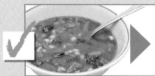

Campbell's Select Harvest Light Vegetable Beef and Barley Soup

SERVING: 1 cup
CALORIES: 80
FAT: 1.5 g
CARBS: 14 g
FIBER: 4 g
SUGAR: 3 g
SODIUM: 480 mg
PROTEIN: 5 g

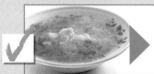

Chicken Soup with Wild Rice and Vegetables

SERVING: 1 cup
CALORIES: 100
FAT: 1 g
CARBS: 16 g
FIBER: 0.5 g
SUGAR: 1 g
SODIUM: 870 mg
PROTEIN: 5 g

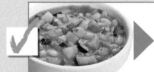

Low-Sodium Vegetable Soup

SERVING: 1 cup
CALORIES: 160
FAT: 2.2 g
CARBS: 29.8 g
FIBER: 5.2 g
SUGAR: 10.6 g
SODIUM: 947 mg
PROTEIN: 5.4 g

Give It a Try!

Reduced-sodium miso soup
25 calories, 1 g fat, 3 g carbs

Chicken and wild rice soup
80 calories, 4 g fat, 9 g carbs

Broth-based butternut squash soup
90 calories, 2 g fat, 16 g carbs

Hate the idea of giving up that creamy texture? Modify your soup with low-fat yogurt, milk, tofu or even mashed potato – you'll get the thick, rich texture without the additional fat.

Look for soups that contain extra-lean protein (chicken, fish or lean beef) and added fiber (sweet potatoes or legumes) for more nutritional power.

"An innocent-looking bowl can be a diet downfall."

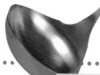

KICK IT

SERVING: 1 cup **CALORIES:** 210 **FAT:** 9 g **CARBS:** 25 g	**FIBER:** 5 g **SUGAR:** 2 g **SODIUM:** 890 mg **PROTEIN:** 7 g	*Chunky New England Clam Chowder*	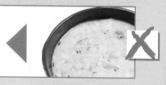

SERVING: 1 cup with cheese and bread **CALORIES:** 310 **FAT:** 14 g	**CARBS:** 35 g **FIBER:** 3 g **SUGAR:** 9 g **SODIUM:** 2,400 mg **PROTEIN:** 17 g	*Baked French Onion Soup*	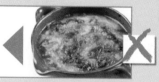

SERVING: 1 cup **CALORIES:** 203 **FAT:** 13.6 g **CARBS:** 15.1 g	**FIBER:** 0.5 g **SUGAR:** 9.3 g **SODIUM:** 918 mg **PROTEIN:** 6.1 g	*Cream of Mushroom Soup*	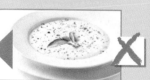

SERVING: 1 cup **CALORIES:** 200 **FAT:** 8 g **CARBS:** 21 g	**FIBER:** 4 g **SUGAR:** 4 g **SODIUM:** 800 mg **PROTEIN:** 11 g	*Chunky Fully Loaded Turkey Pot Pie Soup*	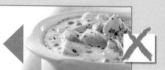

Ditch These Too!

Potato and bacon soup	Lobster bisque soup	Cambell's Fiesta Nacho Cheese soup
170 calories, 7 g fat, 19 g carbs	*260 calories, 18 g fat, 14 g carbs*	*240 calories, 16 g fat, 20 g carbs*

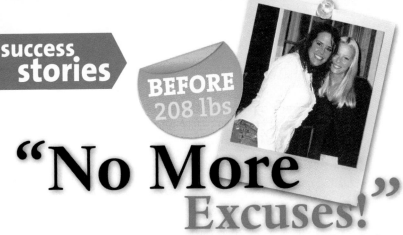

BEFORE
208 lbs

"No More
Excuses!"

At 208 lbs, Beth Peshia used excuses to avoid training and eating properly – till her graduation pictures finally motivated her enough to change for good!

BY WENDY MORLEY

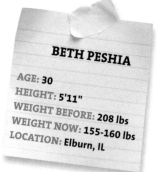

BETH PESHIA

AGE: 30
HEIGHT: 5'11"
WEIGHT BEFORE: 208 lbs
WEIGHT NOW: 155-160 lbs
LOCATION: Elburn, IL

What do family barbecues and housework have in common? They were both excuses for why Beth Peshia couldn't manage to exercise or eat right. When it was time for Beth to work out, she would tell herself that she had too much laundry to do or that she was tired and needed to rest. When she was tempted to eat poorly, she'd tell herself that she'd eat less for the rest of the week or work out more the next day to make up for it.

A PICTURE TRUMPS A THOUSAND EXCUSES

Her excuses came to a stop when Beth saw her college graduation pictures. "I was completely disgusted," she says. "Just looking at those pictures inspired me to change my life." Beth began challenging herself to achieve small, obtainable goals. To stay motivated she bought herself clothes just a little too small. Once they fit, she would buy something smaller still. She constantly challenged herself to do a little more and go a little longer.

SUPPORT AT THE GYM

It's lucky for Beth that she did start going to the gym regularly, because that's where she met her husband! He approached her, saying how impressed he was with her commitment, and that he noticed not only her changing body, but also her growing confidence. A bodybuilder, he introduced Beth to weight training. He became Beth's training partner, sticking with her and supporting her through months of dieting and pre-contest training leading up to her first step onto the physique competition stage. She recently took home first place in a national level contest!

BLENDING COMMITMENTS

At one point some of Beth's friends and family were not supportive of her fitness efforts. She had stopped spending as much time with them because of her new lifestyle. She no longer wanted to go to bars, eat out in fast-food restaurants or even join in family barbecues because the food and drinks served at these places did not fit in with her new lifestyle. Eventually, though, Beth realized she could modify her own behavior while spending time with those close to her. She could go out to bars but sip a low-cal beverage, bring her own food to barbecues, request her food cooked "dry" at restaurants and stick to her goals while keeping her friends. "Now, I have a great balance in my life," she says, "and I've actually motivated many of my friends to put down the booze and pick up a weight." Beth found that the keys to her success were to plan ahead and keep herself surrounded by positive people, and those keys opened the door to her new lean body.

AFTER
155 lbs

"My Pick it Kick it"

LUNCH
PICK IT
Grilled salmon salad with light dressing, tons of veggies and almonds
KICK IT
Fried chicken salad with croutons

DINNER
PICK IT
Broiled tilapia with salt-free herb seasoning, spinach, veggies, almonds and brown rice
KICK IT
Red meat and white rice or fries

MY SUCCESS TIP: "I always order a sweet potato at a restaurant — plain, of course!"

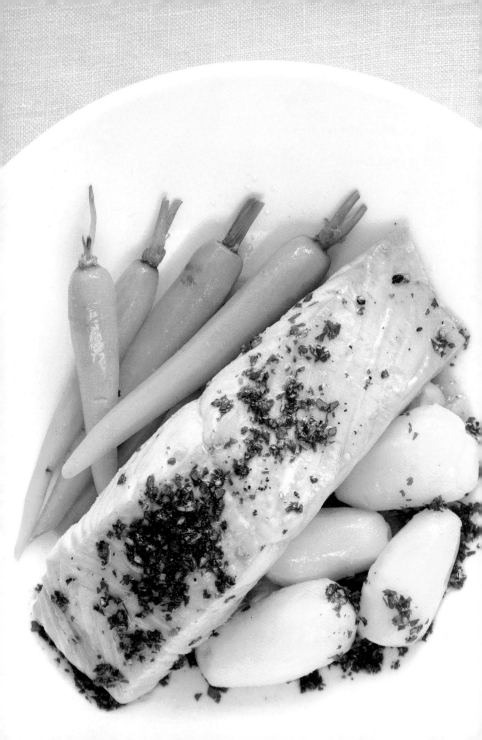

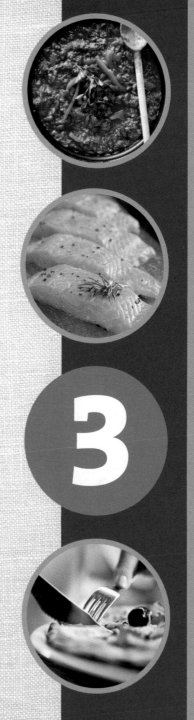

3

Dinner

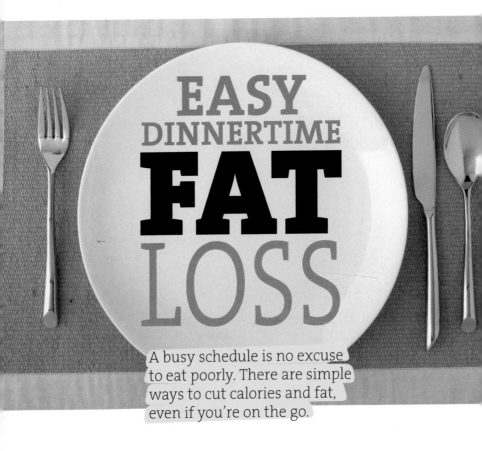

EASY DINNERTIME FAT LOSS

A busy schedule is no excuse to eat poorly. There are simple ways to cut calories and fat, even if you're on the go.

One of my closest friends confided the other day that she can't remember the last time she, her husband and two teenage boys sat down to dinner together. In fact, she admitted to me they eat more often in the car than anywhere else.

With two active teenage boys, there are always football practices, tournaments, away games and rides to friends' houses. Little wonder their car almost knows its own way to the drive-thru. Sadly, her youngest boy has recently been diagnosed with diabetes, a product of the drive-thru lifestyle.

"Don't be badgered into allowing technology to control you – insist on a dinner time and then plan for it."

When I was growing up, a sit-down dinner was a given. Although my dad worked late most evenings, my mother insisted that we all gather around the dinner table for the final meal of the day. And so every evening we'd sit down to dinner, grumbling about how it interfered with our favorite television shows, phone calls from friends or basketball practices. But my mother was adamant; the same way she kept television out of the living room where "conversation takes precedence," she was uncompromising when it came to dinnertime.

When I had my own two kids, I found myself following in my mother's footsteps. If the phone rang, we let it ring. No IM; no texting. Kate and Drew were encouraged to ask questions and let us in on their day. Any interruptions were discouraged. Although I'm not as formal as my mother and never used china for the Sunday meal, our dinners together became an integral part of our daily routines.

Increasingly, research is telling us that the sit-down family dinner isn't just a cute outmoded concept. In fact, it's clearly helpful to the mental and physical health of our families. Teenagers who eat with their families fewer than three times a week are more likely to turn to alcohol, tobacco and drugs than those who eat with them five times a week, according to findings from the National Center on Addiction and Substance Abuse (CASA) at Columbia University (published in the Sunday *New York Times*, October 3, 2009). In the same article, *The Times* cited the NPD Group, a market research firm, as determining that women are responsible for about 80 percent of a family's meals.

I am convinced that all of us, no matter how busy we are, can make time for that one meal of the day – at least a few times a week if not every day. Even if dinner isn't always given the same time slot or length, we have to protect dinnertime as a social glue – one that can bind us to one another in so many intangible ways.

The solution? Don't be badgered into allowing technology to control you – insist on a dinner time and then plan for it. On Sunday afternoons, I spend time chopping veggies and grilling chicken, putting it away in portions for the upcoming week. I make large salads ahead of time, keeping tomatoes separate so they don't ooze and then putting it all together when I come home late after work. And when life gets in the way and I have to pick up sushi or a pizza, I don't beat myself up. If I choose the right kind of pizza or sushi – and in the right portions – these dishes can be as much fun to gather around as any home-cooked meal. Plus, eating this way will help you lose weight – so no more excuses!

PICK IT

Nutritional Value	
SERVING	1 slice
CALORIES	192
FAT	9.9 g
CARBS	16.7 g
FIBER	1.3 g
SUGAR	1.9 g
SODIUM	366 mg
PROTEIN	8.9 g

MAKE IT BETTER

Start your meal with salad to save 100 calories from your second course.

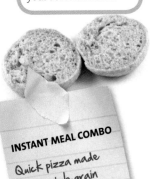

INSTANT MEAL COMBO

Quick pizza made with a whole grain English muffin, ¼ cup tomato sauce and 1 oz part-skim mozzarella cheese, broiled in the oven plus a side salad with 1 Tbsp vinaigrette.

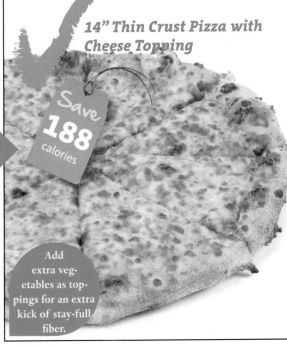

14" Thin Crust Pizza with Cheese Topping

Save **188** calories

Add extra vegetables as toppings for an extra kick of stay-full fiber.

Give It a Try!

Amy's pizza – roasted vegetable
270 calories, 9 g fat, 42 g carbs

Kashi frozen pizza
260 calories, 9 g fat, 29 g carbs

Whole Foods 365 pizza – tomato/pesto
300 calories, 13 g fat, 32 g carbs

Say What?

RESTAURANT MEALS are 15 percent higher in saturated fats and contain 20 percent more fat in general than home-cooked meals. *— US Department of Agriculture*

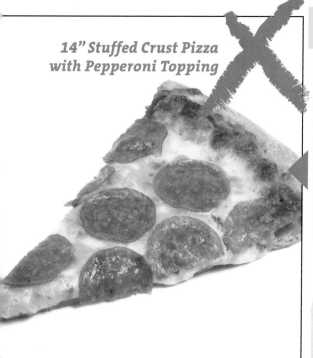

14" Stuffed Crust Pizza with Pepperoni Topping

KICK IT

Nutritional Value	
SERVING	1 slice
CALORIES	380
FAT	18 g
CARBS	39 g
FIBER	2 g
SUGAR	5 g
SODIUM	1,060 mg
PROTEIN	16 g

850

The calories in one 6" Meat Lover's Personal Pan Pizza. Increase your fat loss by choosing a meatless pizza. Add veggies and order a thin crust.

Ditch These Too!

Red Baron frozen pizza – sausage and pepperoni
350 calories, 18 g fat, 33 g carbs

Dipping sauce
250 calories, 28 g fat, 0 carbs

Cheese breadsticks
180 calories, 7 g fat, 20 g carbs

Try This

Toppings of mushrooms and chicken provide a significant amount of tummy-flattening potassium, perfect for balancing the slightly high sodium content from pizza dough.

YES YOU CAN

Grab a training partner. Research shows that when it comes to exercise adherence, you're far more likely to be consistent when someone else is counting on you. Additionally, the spirited competition and support will help you maximize your workout efforts, leading to a stronger and sexier-looking you.

PICK IT

Nutritional Value

SERVING	3 oz
CALORIES	84
FAT	0.9 g
CARBS	0 g
FIBER	0 g
SUGAR	0 g
SODIUM	191 mg
PROTEIN	17.8 g

Plain Sautéed Shrimp

Love This!
(I keep a bag of frozen shrimp on hand for quick protein-packed dinners!)

Save 122 calories

Shrimp is a great source of protein that is just as tasty in salads, in pasta or on its own.

BONUS!

Shrimp is a source of selenium, vitamin D and vitamin B12 – three nutrients Americans are often deficient in.

≫ FAST FACT

Just two alcoholic drinks at dinner can reduce your body's ability to metabolize fat by as much as 73 percent!

Give It a Try!

Sautéed Tiger shrimp
70 calories, 1 g fat, 0 carbs

Baked salmon (4 oz)
200 calories, 9.3 g fat, 0 carbs

Baked halibut (4 oz)
158 calories, 3.3 g fat, 0 carbs

YES YOU CAN Eat better and work out ... at home! Create at-home workouts with push-ups, squats, sit-ups, chair dips and other body-weight exercises. Then grab a clean meal, all without leaving the comfort of your own home. Great for days when you just can't make it to the gym!

Breaded, Fried Shrimp

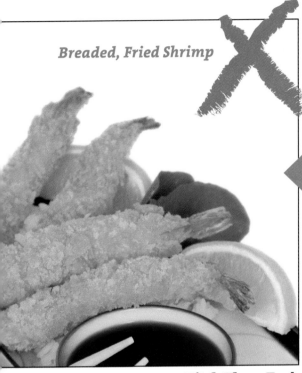

KICK IT

Nutritional Value	
SERVING	3 oz
CALORIES	206
FAT	10.5 g
CARBS	9.8 g
FIBER	0.3 g
SUGAR	0 g
SODIUM	293 mg
PROTEIN	18.2 g

Try This

Eat protein-rich foods at least three times per day. Adequate protein will help you feel full for longer, plus it will help prevent some muscle catabolism as you lose weight. Most women should aim for 80 to 100 grams of protein each day.

Ditch These Too!

Breaded, fried scallops
183 calories, 9.3 g fat, 8.6 g carbs

Breaded, fried oysters
173 calories, 11.1 g fat, 10.2 g carbs

Frozen breaded fish sticks (3 sticks)
209 calories, 11.2 g fat, 17.7 g carbs

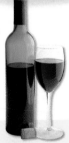

Say What?

AFTER A long day, it's easy to reach for a big meal and a glass of wine, but beware! Natalie Digate Muth, MD, MPH says: "Many physically active women stall their nutrition progress by 'rewarding' themselves after a long day or hard workout with a food binge." You should be wary of wine too, since not only is it full of empty calories, but it may increase your appetite and lower your inhibitions, making you less likely to stick to your food plan.

PICK IT

Nutritional Value

SERVING	1 salad
CALORIES	180
FAT	6 g
CARBS	10 g
FIBER	4 g
SUGAR	5 g
SODIUM	860 mg
PROTEIN	23 g

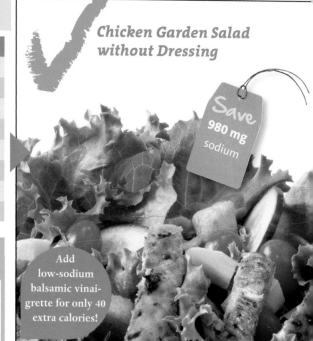

Chicken Garden Salad without Dressing

Save 980 mg sodium

Add low-sodium balsamic vinaigrette for only 40 extra calories!

MAKE IT BETTER

Feel like chicken tonight? Fire up some chicken breasts and tell the legs and thighs to take a hike!

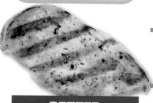

BETTER STILL

Shed the skin on your chicken and you'll feel better showing a little of your own in a slinky dress. Remove the skin after cooking for best flavor.

Give It a Try!

Spinach salad with plain cooked shrimp (3 oz) (spinkle of lemon for dressing)
165 calories, 2.9 g fat, 14 g carbs

Greek salad with pita
283 calories, 5.5 g fat, 50 g carbs

Spinach salad with raspberries
91 calories, 2.1 g fat, 16.3 g carbs

YES YOU CAN

Go green! Double up on veggies and then eat them first, before diving into the rest of your meal.

KICK IT

Chicken Caesar Salad

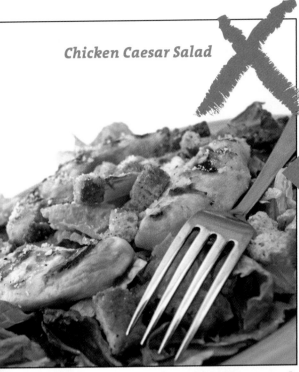

Nutritional Value	
SERVING	1 salad
CALORIES	930
FAT	71 g
CARBS	28 g
FIBER	0.6 g
SUGAR	0 g
SODIUM	1,840 mg
PROTEIN	43 g

FATTER, NOT FITTER

We may feel virtuous because we ate a salad for dinner, but creamy dressings such as Caesar and ranch often pack on more fat and calories than an order of fries.

Ditch These Too!

Egg salad with mayonnaise and onion
370 calories, 32 g fat, 4 g carbs

Ham salad with croutons
366 calories, 10.6 g fat, 44 g carbs

Potato salad with mayonnaise
200 calories, 10 g fat, 24 g carbs

Try This

Be colorful with your fruits and vegetables. Give some excitement to your palate and pack more vitamins onto your plate. The greater the color combination of your vegetables, the higher your intake of antioxidants, which reduce cell damage, improve vision, aid neurological function and strengthen your immune system in general. They'll also help you meet your daily quota of fiber intake.

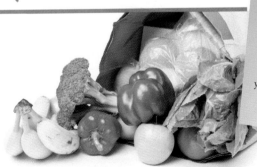

Tuna Roll

Nutritional Value	
SERVING	10 oz
CALORIES	461
FAT	9 g
CARBS	64 g
FIBER	2 g
SUGAR	13 g
SODIUM	906 mg
PROTEIN	23 g

Save
454 mg
sodium

CHOOSE SUSHI WITHOUT SAUCES AND NOT FRIED.

Give It A Try!

☑ **Sashimi (Hamachi)**
122 calories, 1.1 g fat, 0 carbs

☑ **Spicy salmon salad**
180 calories, 8 g fat, 20 g carbs

☑ **Low-sodium miso soup**
40 calories, 1.2 g fat, 5.3 g carbs

Tuna Roll

Ready in 20 minutes •
Makes 4 servings

- 2 cups short-grained brown rice
- 1 tbsp seasoned rice wine vinegar
- 4 sheets nori
- 1 avocado, sliced thinly
- 1 English cucumber, seeded and sliced thinly lengthwise
- 1 lb sashimi-grade tuna fillet, sliced into long chunks

1. Add vinegar to cooked rice and toss to coat. Set aside.

2. Place plastic wrap over a rolling mat. Lay one sheet of nori, shiny side down, on mat. Add one cup of rice, pressing it gently until it covers all the nori. Place remaining ingredients in a horizontal line down the middle, overlapping if necessary.

3. Starting from the end closest to you, roll the mat over itself, making sure to remove the plastic wrap from the roll, until you get to the end. When you've completed your rolls, moisten a sharp knife and cut each roll into about six pieces.

Try This!

Don't like the idea of sushi? Try some ceviche – seafood "cooked" in citrus.

SUSHI

Bite-sized sushi looks so lean and harmless, but not all sushi is created equal.

- A 10-ounce sushi tempura roll or crunchy shrimp roll tops 500 calories and 10 to 20 fat grams.
- White sushi rice adds empty calories.
- You'll even need to watch for items like eel and avocado; they're okay in moderation but contain a lot of fat.

Keep it simple by ordering tuna, salmon or cucumber rolls. Better still – the sashimi platter. You'll avoid the fried batter and benefit from the heart-healthy omega-3 fats in the fish.

QUICK & EASY

Have some edamame as an appetizer while you wait for your sushi. Go easy on the salt, though!

ALL YOU! Schedule a massage. It will help your muscles respond more readily to your training efforts. More importantly, it will relax your muscles, your mind and your spirit. And it will lower your cholesterol levels!

KICK IT

Crunchy Shrimp Roll

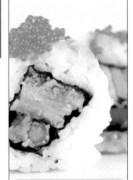

Nutritional Value

SERVING	10 oz
CALORIES	521
FAT	20 g
CARBS	60 g
FIBER	5 g
SUGAR	16 g
SODIUM	1,360 mg
PROTEIN	19 g

Ditch These Too!

Tempura (fried shrimp and veggies)
447 calories, 20.3 g fat, 32.6 g carbs

Beef teriyaki
249 calories, 14.5 g fat, 2.5 g carbs

Regular miso soup
40 calories, 1.2 g fat 5.3 g carbs, 750 mg sodium

SODIUM ALERT!

PICK IT

Nutritional Value

SERVING	1 cup
CALORIES	190
FAT	1 g
CARBS	35 g
FIBER	10 g
SUGAR	6 g
SODIUM	780 mg
PROTEIN	11 g

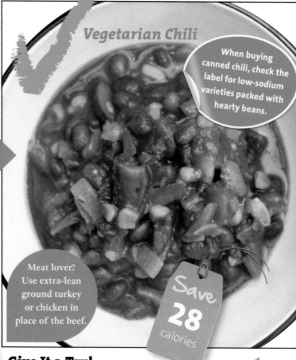

Vegetarian Chili

When buying canned chili, check the label for low-sodium varieties packed with hearty beans.

Meat lover? Use extra-lean ground turkey or chicken in place of the beef.

Save 28 calories

Try This

Combat daily stress with consistent but varying workouts. You'll function better under pressure than those who don't hit the gym.

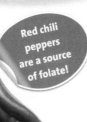

Red chili peppers are a source of folate!

Give It a Try!

Vegetarian chili with extra vegetables
224 calories, 1 g fat, 43 g carbs   ✓

Vegetarian chili with bulgar and black beans
276 calories, 2 g fat, 48 g carbs   ✓

Seafood chili with tomatoes and leeks
363 calories, 5.5 g fat, 38.3 g carbs   ✓

TOP CHOICE! *Chili Peppers*

Chili peppers don't just add an intense flavor kick to any meal, this potent vegetable will also curb your appetite and reduce your fat intake. A little goes a long way – you need only one tablespoon of chopped red or green chili pepper to boost your metabolism. Eat a spicy meal today!

SEASON IT
Add chili peppers to your fat-burning breakfast of egg whites and you'll start burning fat from the start of your day.

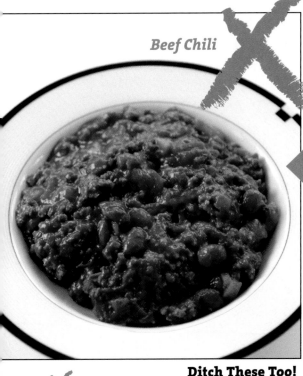

Beef Chili

KICK IT

Nutritional Value	
SERVING	1 cup
CALORIES	218
FAT	7.5 g
CARBS	24.8 g
FIBER	7.5 g
SUGAR	4.5 g
SODIUM	833 mg
PROTEIN	14.3 g

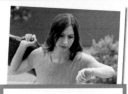

EXCUSE BUSTED

I don't have time to work out or cook healthy meals.

Taking 20 minutes weekly to plan workouts and meals (including healthy take-out options — see chapter five), will not only save the brainwork when you're in a rush, it will save you time in the long run. Make sure to plan some healthy leftovers!

Ditch These Too!

Chili with sausage and cheese
306 calories, 21 g fat, 15 g carbs

Quizno's bread bowl chili
760 calories, 22 g fat, 107 g carbs

Beef chili and cornbread
418 calories, 15 g fat, 52.8 g carbs

YES YOU CAN

Eat more. Consume six small meals throughout the day to control your caloric intake. You'll give your body more fuel and you'll never overstuff yourself out of hunger.

PICK IT

Nutritional Value

SERVING	1 cup with 1 tsp oil
CALORIES	88
FAT	4 g
CARBS	11.4 g
FIBER	4.1 g
SUGAR	2.7 g
SODIUM	52 mg
PROTEIN	4.6 g

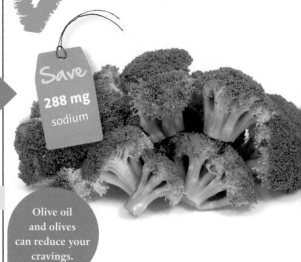

Broccoli, Sautéed with Olive Oil and Garlic

Save
288 mg
sodium

Olive oil and olives can reduce your cravings.

BONUS!

Glutathione
is a powerful but rare antioxidant found in asparagus, broccoli and zucchini.

 FAST FACT

In March 2009, UCLA researchers found a naturally occurring compound in broccoli that may help protect against respiratory conditions such as asthma.

Give It a Try!

Sautéed green beans and carrots with dill
64 calories, 3 g fat, 9 g carbs

Sautéed Brussels sprouts with sliced almonds
87 calories, 5 g fat, 9 g carbs

Roasted yellow and red peppers with salsa
44 calories, 0 fat, 9 g carbs

YES YOU CAN Sign up for a consultation with a registered nutritionist, even if you're already eating clean. Sometimes a professional can see things you might miss and offer valuable insight.

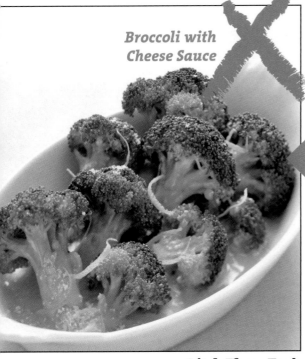

Broccoli with Cheese Sauce

KICK IT

Nutritional Value	
SERVING	1 cup
CALORIES	106
FAT	7 g
CARBS	9 g
FIBER	3 g
SUGAR	0 g
SODIUM	340 mg
PROTEIN	3 g

Try This
Pair your protein with a cup or two of cruciferous vegetables such as bok choy, Brussels sprouts, cauliflower, kale or broccoli to stay healthy, strong and lean.

Ditch These Too!
Deep fried onion rings
255 calories, 11.3 g fat, 36.9 g carbs

Potato wedges with bacon and cheddar cheese
760 calories, 52 g fat, 53 g carbs

Fried zucchini
330 calories, 18 g fat, 36 g carbs

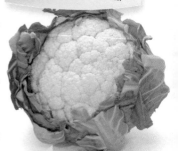

BONUS!

Broccoli is a great source of vitamin C, which makes it an excellent immunity-boosting food. It's also rich in folate and iron and is a good source of calcium, making it a health powerhouse for women.

PICK IT

Nutritional Value

SERVING	8 oz
CALORIES	393
FAT	11.3 g
CARBS	0 g
FIBER	0 g
SUGAR	0 g
SODIUM	93 mg
PROTEIN	68.2 g

A BETTER CHOICE

Use bison in place of beef in fajitas, tacos or burgers – anywhere you would normally eat beef.

TIP Downsize meat portions by one ounce and you'll shave off 50 calories.

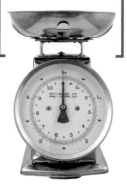

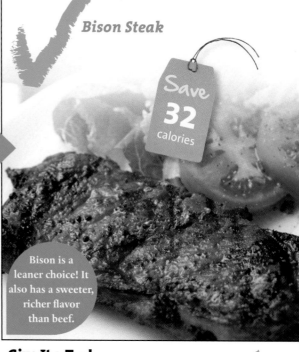

Bison Steak

Save
32
calories

Bison is a leaner choice! It also has a sweeter, richer flavor than beef.

Give It a Try!

Grilled steak (4 oz) with fresh corn salad
307 calories, 10 g fat, 30 g carbs

Grilled buffalo steak (4 oz) with plain baked potato and salsa
303 calories, 2 g fat, 36 g carbs

Grilled steak salad with peppers
135 calories, 15 g fat, 2.5 g carbs

YES YOU CAN Stop eating two to three hours before bedtime. No late dinners!

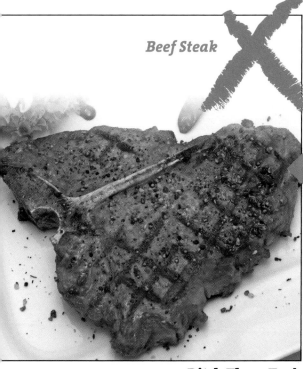

Beef Steak

KICK IT

Nutritional Value	
SERVING	8 oz
CALORIES	425
FAT	14.9 g
CARBS	0 g
FIBER	0 g
SUGAR	0 g
SODIUM	142 mg
PROTEIN	68.5 g

ALL YOU!

Incorporate rest and recovery into your training plan. Muscles don't grow in the gym – they grow in bed. Your muscles and nervous system need time to recover fully, so make sure you leave at least 48 hours between workouts for the same bodypart. On an active rest day, try an activity for fun – yoga, pilates or playing frisbee. Give yourself at least one complete day off from physical activity each week, and take a full week's rest once every six weeks to avoid overtraining and to maintain long-term motivation.

Ditch These Too!

Bacon-wrapped filet mignon
376 calories, 29 g fat, 0 carbs

Peppered New York strip steak (4 oz) and baked potato with sour cream
415 calories, 15 g fat, 35 g carbs

Extra large T-bone steak (16 oz) with gravy
660 calories, 23 g fat, 6 g carbs

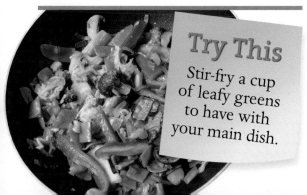

Try This

Stir-fry a cup of leafy greens to have with your main dish.

Stir-Fried Chicken
with Veggies and Steamed Rice

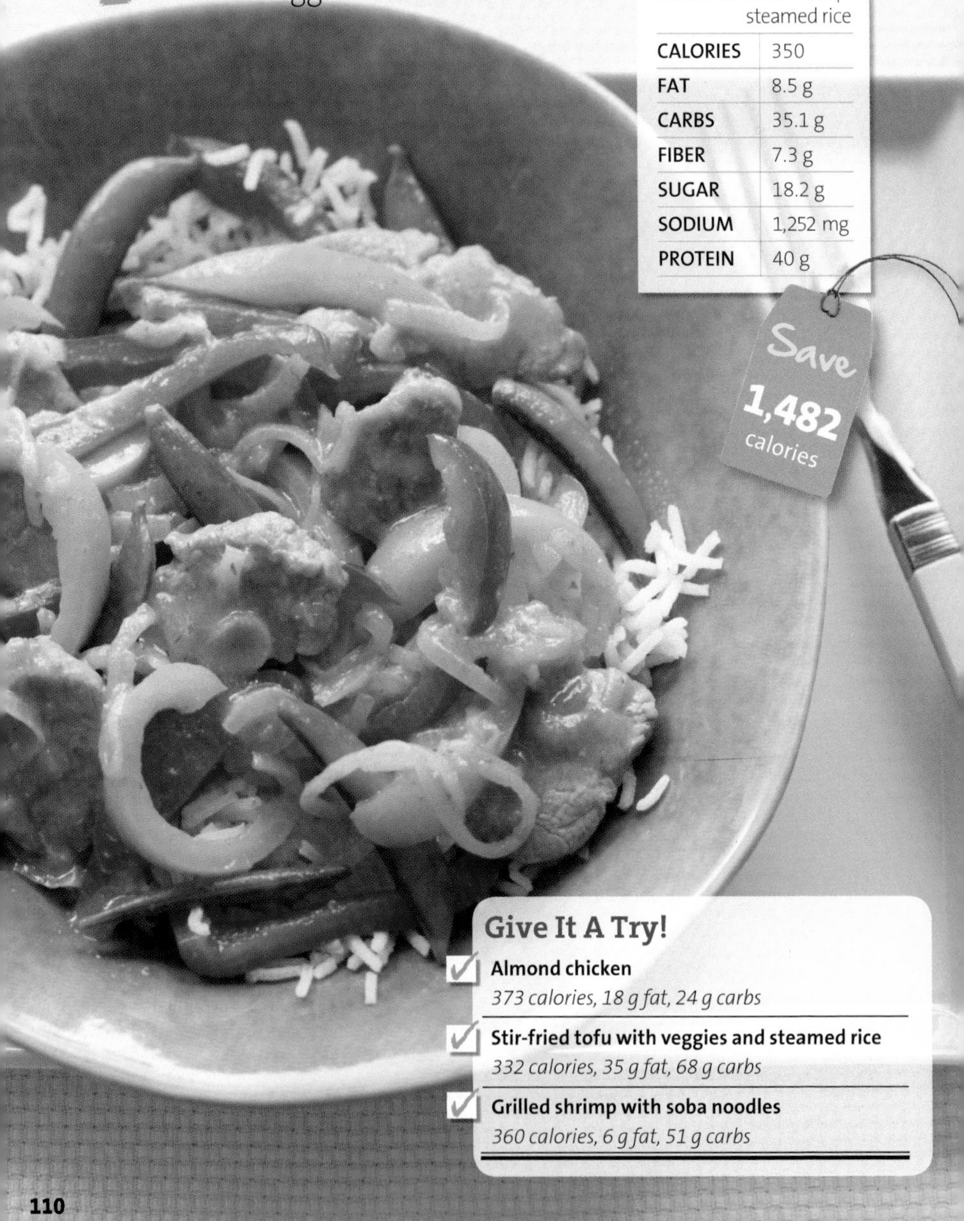

Nutritional Value	
SERVING	5 oz + 1 cup steamed rice
CALORIES	350
FAT	8.5 g
CARBS	35.1 g
FIBER	7.3 g
SUGAR	18.2 g
SODIUM	1,252 mg
PROTEIN	40 g

Save
1,482
calories

Give It A Try!

☑ **Almond chicken**
373 calories, 18 g fat, 24 g carbs

☑ **Stir-fried tofu with veggies and steamed rice**
332 calories, 35 g fat, 68 g carbs

☑ **Grilled shrimp with soba noodles**
360 calories, 6 g fat, 51 g carbs

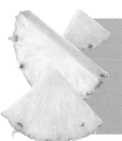

Try This!

When ordering Chinese food, get pineapple chicken (253 calories) instead of sweet and sour chicken (450 calories). You'll get a similar flavor with far fewer calories.

45

Percentage of the American population – nearly half – projected to be obese by 2020, if current trends continue. In fact, according to a study published in the *New England Journal of Medicine*, the U.S. population may not live longer lives because even though smoking rates have declined, more people are overweight.

Minimize restaurant meals.

YES YOU CAN

It's almost impossible to know exactly what you're getting and the portions are large. If you have to eat out, go for quick-serve casual places such as Baja Fresh where nutritional information is available. Check the restaurant's website or menu before you go so you know what to order ahead of time – that way you won't be as tempted to indulge out of sheer hunger. If you really want to be successful at weight loss, you'll need to prepare most of your food at home.

MAKE IT BETTER

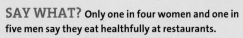

Say no to fried egg rolls and yes to steamed spring rolls.

SAY WHAT? Only one in four women and one in five men say they eat healthfully at restaurants.

– 2007 NEW AMERICAN DINER STUDY BY THE FOOD-SERVICE RESEARCH GROUP RESTAURANTS AND INSTITUTIONS

KICK IT

Sweet and Sour Pork with Fried Rice

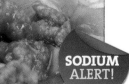

SODIUM ALERT!

Nutritional Value

SERVING	5 oz + 1 cup fried rice
CALORIES	1,832
FAT	91 g
CARBS	188 g
FIBER	9 g
SUGAR	61 g
SODIUM	1,153 mg
PROTEIN	67 g

Ditch These Too!

Pad Thai
560 calories, 20 g fat, 61 g carbs

Pork Vindaloo curry with rice
825 calories, 47.5 g fat, 47.6 g carbs

Deep fried tofu with white rice
512 calories, 23.4 g fat, 56.5 g carbs

PICK IT

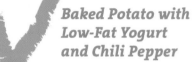

Nutritional Value

SERVING	1 medium
CALORIES	208
FAT	2 g
CARBS	40 g
FIBER	4 g
SUGAR	0 g
SODIUM	232 mg
PROTEIN	8 g

FAST FACT »

One potato provides more than 100 percent of the daily value of vitamin C.

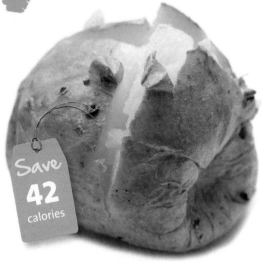

Baked Potato with Low-Fat Yogurt and Chili Pepper

Save **42** calories

Try This

Add some sautéed mushrooms and tomatoes to a baked potato to add some variety and color to your meal!

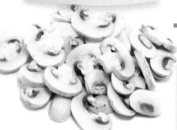

Give It a Try!

Baked potato with dill and low-fat yogurt
293 calories, 1 g fat, 65 g carbs

Baked potato (without skin) with salsa
287 calories, 0 fat, 65 g carbs

Sweet baked potato (with skin) and cinnamon
103 calories, 0.2 g fat, 23.5 g carbs

Say What?

A ONE CUP serving of potato contains only 133 calories! When you eat potatoes you'll keep your heart happy too: they are a good source of potassium, which is a mineral that helps regulate blood pressure.

KICK IT

Baked Potato with Sour Cream and Bacon Bits

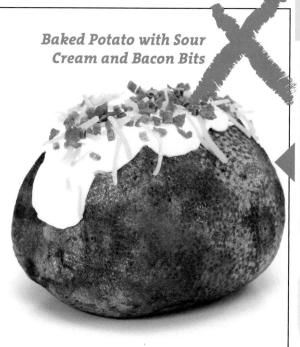

Nutritional Value	
SERVING	1 potato
CALORIES	250
FAT	5 g
CARBS	63 g
FIBER	7 g
SUGAR	4 g
SODIUM	290 mg
PROTEIN	11 g

1 in 10

The number of American women aged 20 or older with diabetes.

Ditch These Too!

Del Monte Savory Sides – potatoes au gratin (1 cup)
160 calories, 5 g fat, 940 mg sodium

Michelina's shepherd's pie
310 calories, 15 g fat, 1,190 mg sodium

Lean Cuisine One Dish Favorites – roasted potatoes with broccoli and chedder
230 calories, 5 g fat, 640 mg sodium

MAKE IT **BETTER**

Try a stuffed potato – cut a cooked potato in half and dig it out, saving the skin. Mix up the mashed potato with one tsp dill, one Tbsp goat cheese and one Tbsp salsa. Stuff it back into the potato skin. Mmmmm!

INSTANT MEAL COMBO

Try a salad Nicoise: new potatoes with chunks of tuna and steamed green beans dressed lightly with oil and vinegar. Add some salad greens.

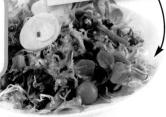

PICK IT

Nutritional Value	
SERVING	1 breast
CALORIES	240
FAT	9 g
CARBS	6 g
FIBER	0 g
SUGAR	1 g
SODIUM	1,462 mg
PROTEIN	35 g

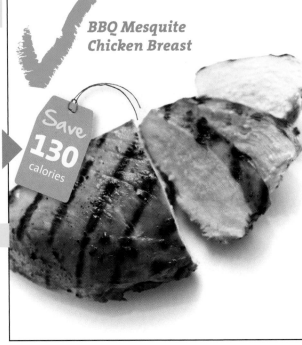

BBQ Mesquite Chicken Breast

Save **130** calories

BONUS!

Four ounces of skinless chicken breast delivers a whopping 121 percent of your daily value of tryptophan, an essential amino acid that promotes nitrogen balance in adults. A positive nitrogen balance ensures continued muscle growth and repair. Moreover, with more than 70 percent of your daily value in niacin (vitamin B3), a four-ounce chicken breast helps your body to fight DNA damage. Niacin is also essential for converting food into energy.

Give It a Try!
Roasted turkey breast
153 calories, 0.8 g fat, 59 mg sodium

Cafe Steamers – grilled chicken marinara
270 calories, 4.5 g fat, 550 mg sodium

Grilled chicken tenders (3 pcs)
261 calories, 18 g fat, 564 mg sodium

BEST BET

Avoid eating chicken with the skin still in place. It may taste great, but it will double the portion's fat content, which will slow the absorption of protein by the body, as well as adding calories and unhealthy fat.

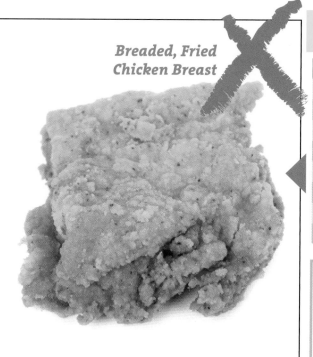

Breaded, Fried Chicken Breast

KICK IT

Nutritional Value	
SERVING	1 breast
CALORIES	370
FAT	21 g
CARBS	7 g
FIBER	0 g
SUGAR	0 g
SODIUM	1,050 mg
PROTEIN	38 g

 FAST FACT

With its unique combination of B-complex vitamins — B3 and B6 — chicken will help your body produce energy.

Ditch These Too!

 Hot and spicy chicken wings
366 calories, 24.6 g fat, 362 mg sodium

 Bacon and cheddar chicken nuggets
302 calories, 21.4 g fat, 655 mg sodium

 Honey barbecue breaded chicken strips
540 calories, 24 g fat, 2,070 mg sodium

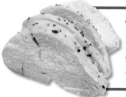

TIP Add boneless, skinless chicken to your weeknight veggie stir-fry for some added protein.

> QUICK & EASY

Chicken Topping
Top grilled chicken breasts with salsa and avocado to add a dash of spice and flavor to your meal.

Breaded Chicken
Mix two cups yogurt with one Tbsp Dijon mustard (or to taste); then dip the chicken breast into the yogurt/mustard mixture before dipping into the breadcrumbs. Bake at 350°F.

PICK IT

Nutritional Value

SERVING	4 oz
CALORIES	111
FAT	1.3 g
CARBS	21.7 g
FIBER	1.2 g
SUGAR	2.5 g
SODIUM	436 mg
PROTEIN	3.7 g

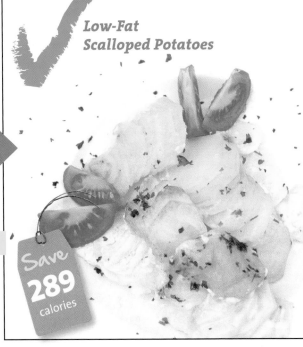

Low-Fat
Scalloped Potatoes

Save
289
calories

BONUS!

As you know, dairy is a rich source of bone-building calcium. What you may not know is that higher calcium intake is associated with lower body-fat levels.

Say What?

THINK YOU might have to cut out potatoes to eat well? Contrary to popular opinion, potatoes are good for you! A medium-sized potato is only 155 calories and is virtually free of sodium and fat. Potatoes are also good sources of complex carbs, vitamin B6 and fiber, and great sources of vitamin C and potassium.

Give It A Try!

Mashed potatoes with low-fat milk
117 calories, 3.8 g fat, 6 mg sodium

Diced new potatoes with chives
45 calories, 0 fat, 280 mg sodium

Baked potato with rosemary and parmesan cheese
160 calories, 1 g fat, 82 mg sodium

> QUICK & EASY

The next time you peel some potatoes, save the skins! Potato skins can make a great side dish or snack during a busy week. Load potato skins with fresh tomatoes, mushrooms, onions or any leftover vegetables for a nutritious, healthy bite between activities.

KICK IT

Cheesy Scalloped Potatoes

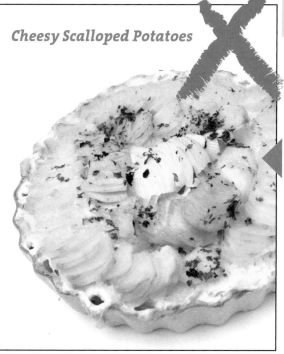

Say What?

POTATOES ARE not only inexpensive, they are the number one vegetable crop in the world.

Ditch These Too!

**Armour Canned Meals –
scalloped potatoes with ham chunks**
240 calories, 10 g fat, 1,090 mg sodium

**Michelina's Signature –
cheddar and broccoli potatoes**
310 calories, 15 g fat, 1,160 mg sodium

Inland Valley – triple cheese potato dish
200 calories, 9 g fat, 390 mg sodium

100

Number of edible varieties of potatoes.

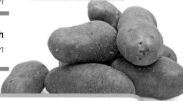

MAKE IT **BETTER**

Replace the cream or high-fat milk in your favorite scalloped potatoes recipe with skim or soy milk. Substitute a low-fat alternative for high-fat cheddar cheese.

MINDFUL EATING

*O*xygen columnist and best-selling author Tosca Reno has a wise piece of advice for all of us who indulge in a little impulse shopping now and again: wait a minute. If you see something that you simply "have to have," wait a minute. If that something still screams at you after a moment's reflection, purchase it.

The same advice applies to eating. Just like impulse shopping, eating mindlessly, or without thought, is a dangerous habit. Maybe you've been so busy all day that you haven't had time to plan your meals and so, on the way home from work, you aim your car into a drive-thru and order a burger and fries. Or perhaps you walk past the food court in the shopping mall and impulsively grab a Chinese take-out, just to tide you over for the afternoon.

The French have a habit of sitting and slowing down to eat – they never even drink a cup of coffee on the run. How overweight are they? It's something to think about. Eating in a rush is all about indulging an urge – and it can be hazardous to both your health and your waistline.

The grab-and-go lifestyle is partly to blame. Research shows that we are devoting less and less time to the art of eating: adults in the United States spend double the amount of time watching television each day (two-and-a-half to three hours) than eating (only one hour and twelve minutes). And let's not forget how much time is spent mindlessly eating in front of the TV! (66 percent of Americans regularly eat in front of the television.) Studies show kids fare no better: students are given only seven to eleven minutes to eat their lunches before they are sent outside to play. – Vangsness, Stephanie, R.D., L.D.N., C.N.S.D, Brigham and Women's Hospital, "Mastering the Mindful Meal"

When your mind is not fully engaged in eating, your digestive process is 30 to 40 percent less effective. Being aware of what's on your plate and savoring the actual experience of eating is called mindful eating. Harvard dietician Stephanie Meyers, R.D., L.D.N., C.N.S.D. advocates mindful eating and suggests you try this exercise with a friend:

1. Take one bite of an apple and close your eyes. Don't start chewing yet.
2. Focus on the apple, instead of the ideas running through your brain. Notice the texture, taste and temperature of the apple.
3. Begin to chew slowly. Notice each movement of your jaw.
4. Try not to swallow the apple slice. Instead, enjoy the sensations in your mouth.
5. Move the apple to the back of your tongue and throat, then slowly swallow.
6. Take a deep breath and exhale.

MINDFUL MOUTHFULS!

You don't have to eat like this at every meal, but you should make an effort to enjoy the sensation of eating rather than stuffing bites in your mouth without even tasting your food. Here are some other ways you can teach yourself to slow down and eat mindfully at the dinner table:

- Eat with chopsticks
- Eat without the television, a newspaper or the computer
- Eat with a companion: a friend, significant other or family member
- Set parameters: if the phone rings, don't answer it; no texting during meals; the only activity at the table is conversation
- Eat sitting down
- Practice proper portions and make every meal last at least 20 minutes.

Try these extra mindful eating strategies that will have you blasting fat in no time:

- Put down your fork after every bite. You'll allow yourself more time to experience the taste and texture of the food you're eating. Plus, you'll give yourself more time to digest each bite, which will allow you to stop eating once you reach the bite that makes you feel full.
- Try eating with your non-dominant hand. It may seem silly at first, but it's one of the best ways to train yourself to really think about and focus on how and what you're eating.
- Eat only when hungry. If you can only think about one specific food, you're probably experiencing a craving. Take a minute to center yourself before packing your plate.
- Keep a log of how your surroundings impact your eating. Do you eat more in a familiar place? At a specific time of day? Around certain people? Recognize your triggers to eliminate them.

PICK IT

Nutritional Value

SERVING	3 oz
CALORIES	444
FAT	6 g
CARBS	74 g
FIBER	5 g
SUGAR	8 g
SODIUM	271 mg
PROTEIN	19 g

A BETTER CHOICE

Lose the high-fat content of macaroni and cheese and embrace the healthy benefits of this home-style, low-fat Italian American dish.

>> FAST FACT

Research continues to prove the undeniable fat-fighting powers of low-fat dairy foods. In a study published in the journal Nutrition & Metabolism, *participants in the high-dairy consumption group, who ate three servings per day, were actually able to consume more calories without any weight gain.*

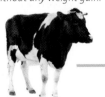

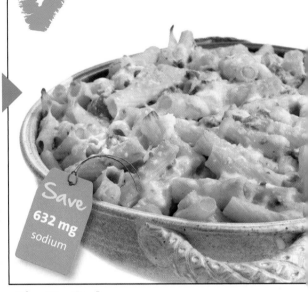

Low-Fat Baked Ziti

Save 632 mg sodium

Give It a Try!

Eden Organic whole grain kamut pasta – diced tomatoes and basil
235 calories, 1.5 g fat, 38.6 g carbs

Whole wheat penne with tomatoes and parmesan cheese
209 calories, 2 g fat, 357 mg sodium

Hodgson Mill whole wheat blend plus flax fettucine
210 calories, 1 g fat, 0 sodium

Say What?

LOW-FAT RICOTTA CHEESE. While it might not be on your radar – yet – ricotta is a great choice for those ready to expand their horizons beyond cottage cheese and plain yogurt. Whether you use it in a recovery snack, a meal or even as part of a dessert, low-fat ricotta is lean, protein-rich and an excellent source of calcium.

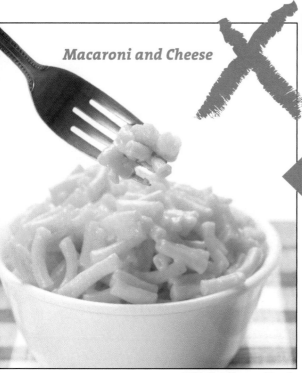

Macaroni and Cheese

KICK IT

Nutritional Value	
SERVING	3 oz
CALORIES	320
FAT	10 g
CARBS	45 g
FIBER	1 g
SUGAR	4 g
SODIUM	903 mg
PROTEIN	12 g

20 million

Number of people suffering from osteoporosis in the United States. Restore a calcium-deficient diet by eating foods rich in the nutrient.

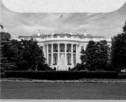

Ditch These Too!

Stouffer's – frozen macaroni and cheese with broccoli
340 calories, 16 g fat, 820 mg sodium

Kraft Macaroni & Cheese dinner
316 calories, 4.3 g fat, 705 mg sodium

Michelina's – frozen cheeseburger mac
350 calories, 12 g fat, 720 mg sodium

≫ FAST FACT

When it comes to dinner, even the President doesn't mess around. No matter what is on his agenda, President Obama always makes time to sit down to dinner every evening at 6PM with his family. In fact, so integral are family dinners to the President, that he insists any night-time duties be scheduled for after 8PM. The family-friendly message is clear – taking time out of a busy day to sit down and eat with the ones you love is a growing trend among American families... even those who live in the White House!

PICK IT

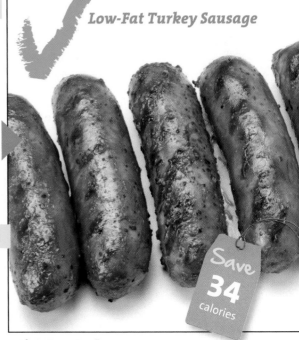

Low-Fat Turkey Sausage

Nutritional Value	
SERVING	4 oz
CALORIES	196
FAT	10.4 g
CARBS	0 g
FIBER	0 g
SUGAR	0 g
SODIUM	665 mg
PROTEIN	23.9 g

Save **34** calories

BONUS!

Turkey is a great source of selenium, a nutrient which is of major importance to human health because of its cancer-preventive properties. Turkey is also a source of more cancer-protective nutrients, the B vitamin niacin and B6. These two B vitamins are important for energy production. Four ounces of turkey supplies 27 percent of your daily need for vitamin B6.

Give It a Try!
Applegate Farms organic sweet Italian sausage
130 calories, 7 g fat, 500 mg sodium

Al Fresco sweet Italian style chicken sausage
130 calories, 7 g fat, 480 mg sodium

Simply the Best veggie dog
90 calories, 5 g fat, 310 mg sodium

≫ FAST FACT
Turkey is an excellent source of protein. A four-ounce serving provides about 65 percent of the daily requirement for protein.

TIP Most nutritionists swear by food journals or diaries, in which you note what you eat throughout the day for at least a week. Keeping a food journal helps you track what you're eating, makes you accountable and makes it easier for you to identify areas for improvement.

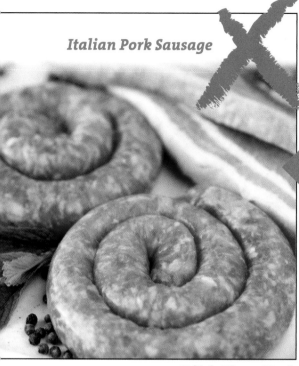

Italian Pork Sausage

Nutritional Value	
SERVING	4 oz
CALORIES	230
FAT	18.3 g
CARBS	2.9 g
FIBER	0.1 g
SUGAR	0.6 g
SODIUM	809 mg
PROTEIN	12.8 g

A BETTER CHOICE

We all have our favorite treats. Cutting out your indulgences entirely usually leads to an early relapse in unhealthy eating. There's no problem with allowing yourself a treat now and then, but keep an eye on the frequency and the quantity.

Ditch These Too!

Stouffer's Swedish meatballs
560 calories, 27 g fat, 1,150 mg sodium

Hillshire Farm beef smoked sausage
210 calories, 18 g fat, 560 mg sodium

7-Eleven Big Bite hot dog (no bun)
480 calories, 45 g fat, 1,510 mg sodium

Say What?

MORE THAN HALF the calories in most regular sausages come from fat, with summer sausages as some of the fattiest. A good rule of thumb is to not reach for the thickest sausage – they'll pack on the fat and calories!

MAKE IT **BETTER**

When using meat in cooking, treat it as a complement to a meal of vegetables, grains or legumes instead of the main feature. Portions of meat should not be more than three to four ounces.

PICK IT

Nutritional Value

SERVING	1 cup cooked
CALORIES	218
FAT	1.6 g
CARBS	45.8 g
FIBER	3.5 g
SUGAR	0 g
SODIUM	2 mg
PROTEIN	4.5 g

30%

Women who eat an average of two to three servings of whole grains a day are 30 percent less likely to develop type 2 diabetes than women who rarely eat whole grains.
– Harvard School of Public Health

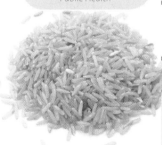

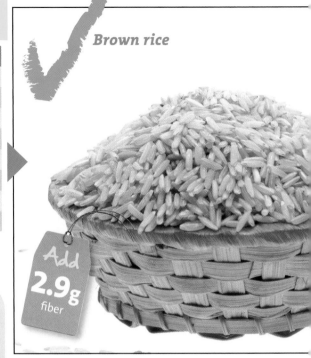

Brown rice

Add **2.9g** fiber

Give It a Try!

Kashi Whole Grain Pilaf – fiery fiesta
210 calories, 5 g fat, 400 mg sodium

Rice-A-Roni – whole grain chicken and herb
260 calories, 8 g fat, 760 mg sodium

Eden Organic rice & beans
220 calories, 2 g fat, 270 mg sodium

Say What?

THE CONVERSION of brown rice into white rice eliminates 67 percent of the vitamin B3, 80 percent of the vitamin B1, 90 percent of the vitamin B6, half of the manganese, half of the phosphorus, 60 percent of the iron, and all of the dietary fiber and essential fatty acids.

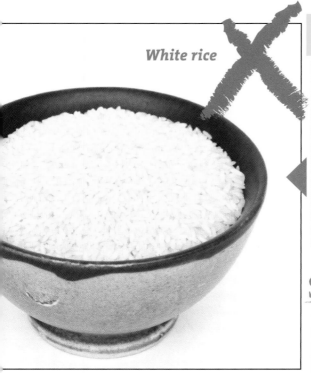

White rice

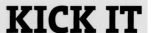

KICK IT

Nutritional Value	
SERVING	1 cup cooked
CALORIES	205
FAT	0.5 g
CARBS	44.6 g
FIBER	0.6 g
SUGAR	0.1 g
SODIUM	2 mg
PROTEIN	4.3 g

Say What?

IT'S THAT TIME of the month! A fluctuation in hormones before and during your menstrual cycle can sabotage even the strictest diet. Estrogen influences our appetite and menstruation causes hormone levels to surge. A study by Dr. Neal Barnard, founder and president of The Physicians Committee for Responsible Medicine (PCRM), found that excess body fat leads to increased estrogen activity, as does a high-fat, low-fiber diet. Conversely, a low-fat, high-fiber diet decreased estrogen levels and PMS symptoms overall.

Ditch These Too!
Rice-A-Roni – herb and butter
310 calories, 9 g fat, 1,160 mg sodium

Rice-A-Roni – chicken
310 calories, 9 g fat, 1,160 mg sodium

Knorr Rice Sides – herb and butter
500 calories, 8 g fat, 1,680 mg sodium

» FAST FACT

In some areas of the world, the phrase "to eat" means "to eat rice." Rice supplies as much as half of the daily calories for half of the world's population.

PICK IT

Pan Fried Fish
with Oven Fries

Nutritional Value	
SERVING	4 oz + 14 pcs
CALORIES	301
FAT	8 g
CARBS	24 g
FIBER	2 g
SUGAR	0.5 g
SODIUM	165 mg
PROTEIN	33 g

Save **989** calories

Give It A Try!

Healthy Choice – frozen fish dinner with lemon pepper
310 calories, 4.5 g fat, 440 mg sodium

Gorton's classic grilled salmon
100 calories, 3.5 g fat, 310 mg sodium

Water-packed tuna (low sodium)
120 calories, 1 g fat, 200 mg sodium

Fish and Chips

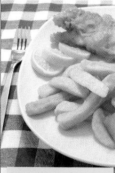

Try This!

If you're eating out, order your fish steamed and your potato baked to cut down on the amount of fat you consume.

BONUS!

When you cook fresh tuna along with its skin, you get the health-promoting omega-3 fatty acids. Another plus: Omega 3s are not stored as readily on your hips. But if you have canned tuna packed in vegetable oil, you miss out on about 50 percent of the omega-3 fats. For the best flavor and nutrition, choose fresh tuna, baked or grilled. If you are reaching for canned tuna, make sure it's water-packed and low-sodium. Remember to monitor your tuna intake to avoid mercury. Have albacore tuna no more than once per week.

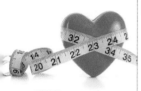

FAST FACT

Worried that eating seafood will raise your blood cholesterol? In fact, the dietary cholesterol found in seafood has little effect on blood cholesterol in most people. Saturated fats and trans fatty acids are the most important factors that raise blood cholesterol.

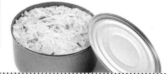

Nutritional Value

SERVING	1 large serving
CALORIES	1,290
FAT	57 g
CARBS	119 g
FIBER	10 g
SUGAR	10 g
SODIUM	2,166 mg
PROTEIN	69 g

Ditch These Too!

✗ **Stouffer's – frozen seafood scampi**
400 calories, 12 g fat, 960 mg sodium

✗ **Seafood cocktail sauce, (¼ cup)**
60 calories, 0 fat, 690 mg sodium

✗ **Breaded fish sticks**
260 calories, 13 g fat, 370 mg sodium

SAY WHAT? If you get moving, you'll benefit even more from eating fish, suggests a study in the *American Journal of Clinical Nutrition*. The study found that the fat-burning effects of fish oil were increased when combined with an aerobic exercise routine in overweight volunteers. A source of lean protein, fish also supply your body with the amino acids it needs to prevent muscle breakdown. So try some mackerel, salmon or sardines the next time you're preparing a meal.

PICK IT

Nutritional Value

SERVING	1 cup
CALORIES	133
FAT	1.6 g
CARBS	30.5 g
FIBER	3.3 g
SUGAR	5.7 g
SODIUM	351 mg
PROTEIN	4.3 g

A BETTER CHOICE

Think that a diet rich in protein and low in carbs is the master plan for building muscle? Think again. A low-carb diet can actually limit your potential if you're not careful. "Some women try to make room for more protein-rich foods by eating fewer fruits, vegetables and other carbohydrate-rich foods that contain certain essential vitamins and minerals (such as vitamins B6 and C) that are needed to reduce muscle inflammation, as well as repair and rebuild muscle," says Jim White, RD, ACSM, national spokesperson for the American Dietetic Association.

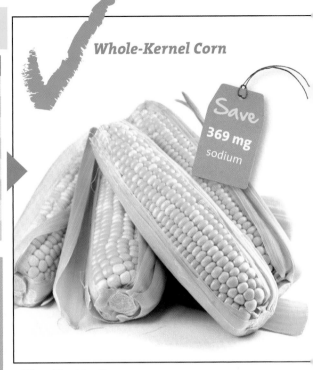

Whole-Kernel Corn

Save
369 mg
sodium

Give It a Try!

Green Giant Frozen Valley Fresh Steamers – broccoli, carrots and cauliflower
45 calories, 1 g fat, 290 mg sodium

Birds Eye – tuscan vegetables in herbed tomato sauce
50 calories, 2 g fat, 180 mg sodium

Baked butternut squash (1 cup)
82 calories, 0 fat, 8 mg sodium

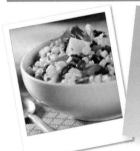

Try This

Add variety to a garden salad by combining whole-kernel corn, tomatoes, chopped green peppers and red kidney beans.

Cream-Style Corn

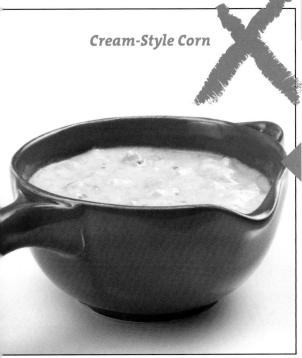

KICK IT

Nutritional Value	
SERVING	1 cup
CALORIES	120
FAT	1 g
CARBS	28 g
FIBER	4 g
SUGAR	14 g
SODIUM	720 mg
PROTEIN	2 g

Ditch These Too!

Birds Eye – pasta and vegetables in creamy cheese sauce
320 calories, 7 g fat, 1,180 mg sodium

Green Giant canned corn niblets
240 calories, 1.5 g fat, 690 mg sodium

S & W candied yams
340 calories, 0 fat, 720 mg sodium, 42 g sugar

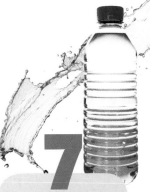

7

The number, when listed at the bottom of a reusable hard-plastic water bottle, that indicates BPA. See it? Toss it.

YES YOU CAN

Ride your bike or walk to work. You'll be more likely to have healthier triglyceride levels and lower cholesterol, according to a new study. Still burning gas instead of calories? Dedicate at least one day a week to alternative transportation and improve your body and the environment at the same time!

PICK IT

Nutritional Value

SERVING	8 oz (3 slices)
CALORIES	477
FAT	8 g
CARBS	48 g
FIBER	9 g
SUGAR	7 g
SODIUM	258 mg
PROTEIN	52 g

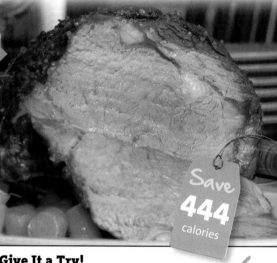

Lean Cut Pot Roast with Veggies and Plain Sweet Potatoes

Save **444** calories

MAKE IT BETTER

Substitute an oven roast with a lean cut pot roast to cut down on fat. Replace side dishes of potatoes and sour cream with veggies and plain sweet potatoes to stock up on the health benefits of fruits and vegetables.

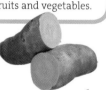

Give It a Try!

Stouffer's – beef pot roast
320 calories, 8 g fat, 1,570 mg sodium ✓

Marie Callender's – slow roasted beef
330 calories, 10 g fat, 970 mg sodium ✓

Lean Cuisine Café Classics – garlic beef and broccoli
170 calories, 6 g fat, 520 mg sodium ✓

Say What?

STUDIES HAVE SHOWN that eating fruits and vegetables can reduce breast cancer recurrence. Researchers from the University of California studied more than 1,550 women previously treated for breast cancer. After five years of follow-up, they found that women with the highest plasma carotenoid concentration, supplied by a high fruit and veggie intake, had a 40 percent reduced risk for breast cancer recurrence over those with lower intake.

KICK IT

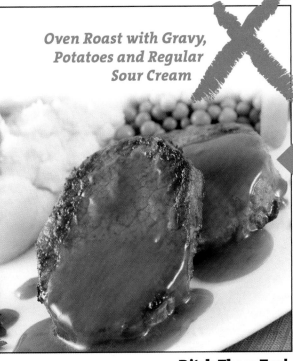

Oven Roast with Gravy, Potatoes and Regular Sour Cream

Nutritional Value	
SERVING	8 oz (3 slices)
CALORIES	921
FAT	51 g
CARBS	43 g
FIBER	5 g
SUGAR	3 g
SODIUM	1,447 mg
PROTEIN	53 g

≫ FAST FACT

It is a myth that you have to cut out red meat to eat well. Instead of excluding red meats completely, choose leaner cuts of beef and pork. For beef, opt for eye of round, top round roast, top sirloin and flank; for pork, go for tenderloin and loin chops.

Ditch These Too!

Banquet beef pot pie
450 calories, 27 g fat, 730 mg sodium

Marie Callender's – beef and broccoli
400 calories, 14 g fat, 1,200 mg sodium

Boston Market – beef sirloin stroganoff and noodles
390 calories, 17 g fat, 780 mg sodium

Try This

When you're shopping for beef, choose cuts labeled "Choice" or "Select" instead of "Prime," which usually has more fat.

DID YOU KNOW?

Comfort foods are popular with most Americans today. Cheap and easy to make, they can be also high in fat and calories. However, pot roast – a lean cut and paired with nutrient-rich veggies and a plain potato with herbs – can be one of the most nutritious comfort foods on the market.

TIP Make it yourself and save on calories and sodium!

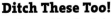

PICK IT

Nutritional Value

SERVING	3 oz
CALORIES	126
FAT	7 g
CARBS	11.9 g
FIBER	1.4 g
SUGAR	1.4 g
SODIUM	161 mg
PROTEIN	2.8 g

> ## QUICK & EASY

Follow this recipe to make healthy, low-fat pasta primavera:

1 lb fettucini or spaghetti
(whole wheat)

1 cup broccoli

1 cup mushrooms, chopped

1 cup ripe olives, pitted

1 cup carrots, peeled, sliced

1 cup artichoke hearts

1 cup zucchini, thickly sliced

⅓ cup olive oil

½ tsp garlic powder

1 tsp dried oregano,
crumbled

1 tsp dried basil, crumbled

½ tsp crushed red pepper

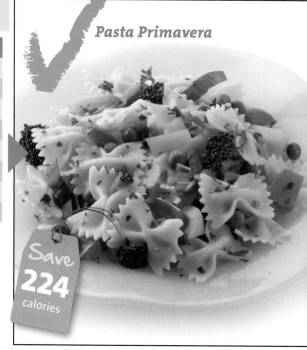

Pasta Primavera

Save
224
calories

Give It a Try!

Bertolli – shrimp and penne primavera
128 calories, 6 g fat, 356 mg sodium

Michelina's – budget gourmet macaroni and cheese
78 calories, 2.1 g fat, 165 mg sodium

Kashi – pesto primavera
87 calories, 3.3 g fat, 225 mg sodium

Cook pasta. Rinse and drain all vegetables; set aside. Drain pasta well and transfer temporarily to serving platter. Heat olive oil in the pan the pasta was cooked in. Stir in garlic powder, oregano, basil and crushed red pepper. Return pasta and all vegetables (well drained) to pan. Toss to coat pasta and vegetables with olive oil/herb mixture. Heat through while tossing frequently. Serve immediately.

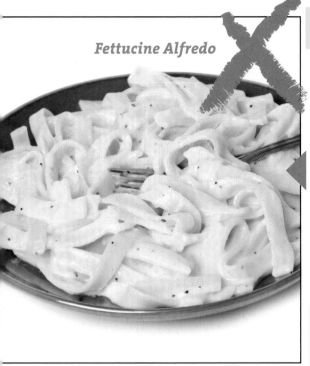

Fettucine Alfredo

KICK IT

Nutritional Value	
SERVING	3 oz
CALORIES	350
FAT	19.8 g
CARBS	35.7 g
FIBER	1.6 g
SUGAR	1.5 g
SODIUM	103 mg
PROTEIN	7.4 g

6

According to the New York State Department of Health's Division of Nutrition, six of the ten leading causes of death in the United States are linked to a poor diet.

Ditch These Too!

Michelina's – fettucine alfredo with chicken and broccoli
109 calories, 3.9 g fat, 240 mg sodium

Banquet – spaghetti and meatballs
120 calories, 5.1 g fat, 282 mg sodium

Stouffer's – chicken Cordon Bleu pasta
330 calories, 15 g fat, 920 mg sodium

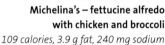

BONUS!

Not only is pasta primavera a low-fat alternative to fettucine alfredo, it is also an excellent source of vitamins K, C and A, and a good source of manganese, dietary fiber and potassium.

Try This

Whole grains contain B vitamins, vitamin E, magnesium, iron and fiber. Look for the word "whole" when shopping for cereals, biscuits, pasta and breads. The new 2005 Dietary Guidelines for Americans recommend that all adults eat at least half their grains as whole grains – that's three to five servings of whole grains a day.

PICK IT

Nutritional Value

SERVING	1 cup
CALORIES	240
FAT	6 g
CARBS	27 g
FIBER	1 g
SUGAR	7 g
SODIUM	880 mg
PROTEIN	21 g

A BETTER CHOICE

Need a quick and easy dinner option? Opt for Hamburger Helper Lasagna, with 240 calories (100 calories from fat) over Hamburger Helper Double Cheese Quesadilla, which packs in 350 calories (110 calories from fat). For an even healthier meal, choose extra lean ground turkey rather than regular ground beef.

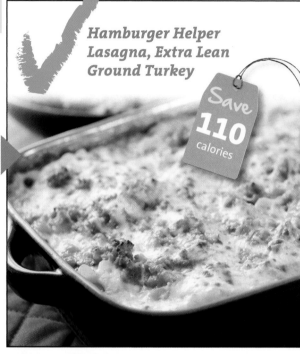

Hamburger Helper Lasagna, Extra Lean Ground Turkey

Save **110** calories

Give It a Try!

Lean Cuisine skillets – chicken primavera
90 calories, 1.3 g fat, 215 mg sodium

Banquet Crockpot Classics – beef pot roast
150 calories, 3.5 g fat, 660 mg sodium

Betty Crocker Chicken Helper – chicken fried rice
250 calories, 9 g fat, 550 mg sodium

YES YOU CAN Grocery shop for healthy food on the run! Reach for pre-cut and washed fresh fruit or vegetables – they can be part of a healthy meal or snack. Go for quick-cooking grains such as fresh pasta, converted rice and couscous to save cooking time. Opt for pre-marinated meat, poultry, fish, kebabs or prawn skewers to cut down on preparation time. Canned beans and lentils are a healthy alternative to meat. Add them to your favourite soups, chilis, pasta sauces or salads.

KICK IT

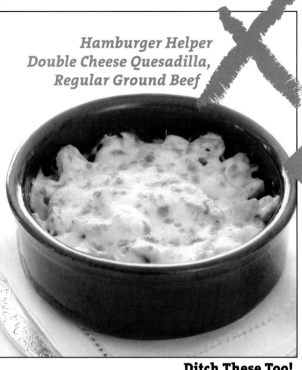

Hamburger Helper Double Cheese Quesadilla, Regular Ground Beef

Nutritional Value

SERVING	1 cup
CALORIES	350
FAT	13 g
CARBS	40 g
FIBER	0.5 g
SUGAR	6 g
SODIUM	840 mg
PROTEIN	21 g

TIP For ground beef recipes, use ground turkey instead. Turkey is lower in fat and works well for burgers and chili.

Ditch These Too!

Bertolli – cheese tortelloni in tomato cream sauce
330 calories, 13 g fat, 1,190 mg sodium

Banquet Crockpot Classics – beef stroganoff and noodles
300 calories, 14 g fat, 800 mg sodium

Betty Crocker Chicken Helper – Mexican cheesy chicken enchilada
330 calories, 7 g fat, 820 mg sodium

TIP Beware when purchasing ground turkey. Regular ground turkey contains nearly 15 grams of fat, while ground turkey breast boasts of only one gram of fat!

Try This

Avoid drinking your calories! According to the Harvard Medical School, eliminating just one sugary soda or high-fat latte can save you 100 or more calories a day. The result? Over a year, avoiding empty calories in liquid form can translate into a 10-lb weight loss.

Your
Pick it
Kick it
Kitchen

A well-stocked kitchen is like a strong core – the foundation of it all.

Fast and easy ways to make the most important room in the house (save the bedroom) meet your fitness needs.

BY JULIE UPTON, MS, RD, AND
CATHERINE BROIHIER, MS, RD

Most of us will be stretching our food budget by eating more meals at home. That's good news because those meals are naturally lower in calories and generally healthier than what we can get from take-out. Plus, you know what's in your pantry, which is more than you can say for the restaurant down the street – making eating clean even easier. Want to make the most out of your meals and snacks? Of course you do, but sometimes keeping your shelves stocked with clean-eating staples just isn't enough. Whip your kitchen into shape and it'll be a whole lot easier to eat clean and maintain your fitness levels. Following are ways to set up your kitchen that will not only inspire you to find your inner chef, but will also have your kitchen practically doing the cooking for you. (Well, almost.)

Simple Clean Eating Tips

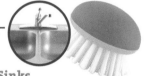

Sinks

Keep a firm scrub brush handy sink-side. Use it to clean firm produce like carrots, cucumber and celery – no special detergents needed.
Clean your sponge. Microwave while damp for one minute or place it in the dishwasher.
Experts do not recommend rinsing raw meat or chicken before cooking – you are just splattering bacteria around.
Dishcloths are eco-friendly but can breed bacteria. Switch cloths each day and wash in hot water.

STORAGE SOLUTIONS
Invest in different sizes and shapes of storage containers; you'll save big bucks and be inspired to enjoy last night's dinner for tomorrow's lunch at work. And keep cooler packs and stainless steel water bottles handy too.

MARKET HEALTHY EATS
Put a bowl of fresh fruit front and center in your kitchen and organize your pantry and refrigerator so that the healthiest foods are at eye level and easy to grab.

FAST FACT
20
The number of seconds you should wash your hands to send bacteria down the drain.
– FIGHTBAC.ORG

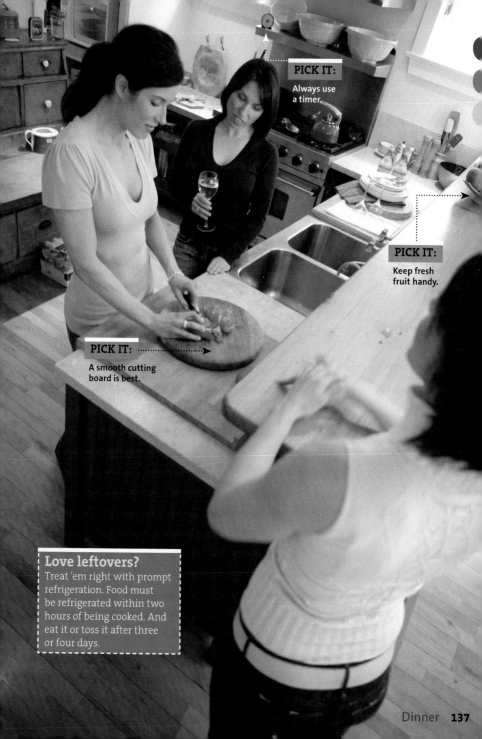

PICK IT:

Always use
a timer.

PICK IT:

Keep fresh
fruit handy.

PICK IT:

A smooth cutting
board is best.

Love leftovers?

Treat 'em right with prompt
refrigeration. Food must
be refrigerated within two
hours of being cooked. And
eat it or toss it after three
or four days.

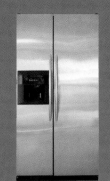

Refrigerator 411

Divide your refrigerator into "eat more often" and "eat less often" areas. Keep a big pitcher of water at eye level as a reminder to drink more every day.

Here are the clean-eating basics that should always be in stock:

- Fresh fruits, vegetables and herbs
- Bagged salad mixes
- Nonfat/low-fat dairy (e.g., milk, cottage cheese, plain yogurt)
- Egg whites, whole eggs
- Cooked lean meat, fish, poultry
- Tofu
- Fortified soy milk
- 100 percent juices
- Olive-oil-based spreads
- Condiments (e.g., mustards, vinegars, lemon and lime juices)

Freezer

- Veggie burgers
- Pork tenderloin
- Whitefish and salmon
- Chicken breasts
- Vegetables and fruits
- Whole grain bread and wraps
- Leftovers

FIT TIP:

Resist using the egg holders in the fridge door! Eggs are more safely stored in their original carton on a shelf where the temperature is cooler and more constant.

FIT TIP:

Flours and grains can be stored in the freezer until needed. Unlike enriched white flour, whole grain flour should stay in an airtight container in the refrigerator because it contains vitamin E and some fat, making it more likely to go rancid before you use all of it.

FIT TIP:

Check labels to determine how food should be stored.

FIT TIP:

Check fridge and freezer temperatures periodically. The fridge shouldn't move the mercury beyond 40°F (5°C) and the freezer should hold steady at a chilly 0°F (-18°C).

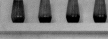

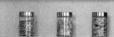

FIT TIP:

Cool air needs to flow. Don't overcrowd your fridge or freezer.

Pantry

A well-stocked pantry is like a strong core; it stabilizes your body to keep you strong. Keep healthy go-to items in stock so you can make meals in minutes and aren't tempted to put in a call to Little Caesars.

In Your Pantry

- Whole grain pasta, bread, breakfast cereal, bulgur, brown rice, quinoa, oatmeal, flaxseeds
- Canned beans, tomato products, low-sodium soups, broths
- Water-packed tuna and salmon
- Lentils

- Salsa, soy sauce
- Olive and canola oil
- Nut butters
- Canola oil vegetable spray
- Dried fruit (e.g., raisins, dried plums)
- Sweet, red and baking potatoes
- Onions

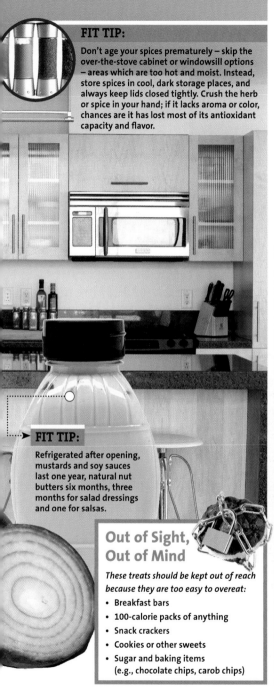

FIT TIP:

Don't age your spices prematurely – skip the over-the-stove cabinet or windowsill options – areas which are too hot and moist. Instead, store spices in cool, dark storage places, and always keep lids closed tightly. Crush the herb or spice in your hand; if it lacks aroma or color, chances are it has lost most of its antioxidant capacity and flavor.

FIT TIP:

Refrigerated after opening, mustards and soy sauces last one year, natural nut butters six months, three months for salad dressings and one for salsas.

Out of Sight, Out of Mind

These treats should be kept out of reach because they are too easy to overeat:

- Breakfast bars
- 100-calorie packs of anything
- Snack crackers
- Cookies or other sweets
- Sugar and baking items
  (e.g., chocolate chips, carob chips)

Cutting Boards

Wood or plastic? The choice is yours. What does matter for cutting board safety are cracks and grooves, which are hotbeds for growing bacteria. Keep cutting board bugs at bay:

- Select a smooth, durable and nonabsorbent board, such as maple or plastic.
- Use two boards – one for raw meats and one for veggies, cheese, fruit, etc.
- Wash countertops, cutting boards (even your sink drain) with a mix of one teaspoon bleach and one quart water.

Five Great Healthy Kitchen Gadgets

Cut your kitchen prep time by keeping these kitchen gizmos within reach.

SALAD SPINNER: The best way to clean greens and worth the space to store it. Smaller "herb" spinners are suitable for solo greens servings.

OIL SPRAYER: Having a refillable, non-aerosol option gives you control over the type of oil you use.

GRATER/ZESTER: Put some zing in your life with lemon, lime and orange zest. It contributes zero calories, but lots of flavor. Plus, it's also good for finely grating hard cheese.

RICE COOKERS: Automatic rice cookers are not only great for cooking rice, but they also make great steel-cut oatmeal that can be ready when you are in the a.m.

STEAMER BASKET: Preserve vitamins by keeping those vegetables out of the water. Microwave steamers are also available and useful for when you're really in a hurry.

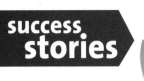
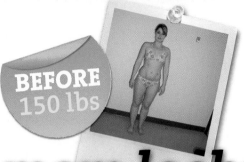

BEFORE
150 lbs

This mom looks
better than ever!

Tammy Stewart ate poorly and didn't exercise, telling herself not to worry about it, because "this is how moms are supposed to look." A photo made her see she'd been kidding herself and she decided she wanted to look good again.

BY WENDY MORLEY

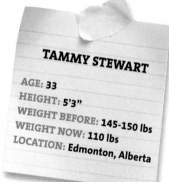

TAMMY STEWART

AGE: **33**
HEIGHT: **5'3"**
WEIGHT BEFORE: **145-150 lbs**
WEIGHT NOW: **110 lbs**
LOCATION: **Edmonton, Alberta**

Like many women, Tammy's weight yo-yo'd for years as she gained and lost the same weight over and over again. But she was comfortable, and even though she ripped the seam in her pants a few times she didn't realize just how much weight she'd actually gained until she saw a picture of herself and finally accepted that she didn't look all that great.

"There will always be people who try to sabotage you with temptation."

NO POST-BABY BODY

Clothes shopping had become a depressing event for Tammy and she decided she didn't want to carry around the extra weight anymore. She was determined to get back to the point at which she felt comfortable in her own skin. When she found out she was having her second child she was more motivated than ever – she did not want to be stuck with a post-baby body again. Sure enough, a few months after her baby was born a friend asked her if she was sure she'd had two kids, because she looked like she'd never had one child, let alone two!

MAKING TIME

The biggest challenge for Tammy throughout her journey has been making time for exercise, in addition to watching what she puts in her mouth. She succeeds by thinking ahead, and planning her day around her workout, leaving no question as to whether or not it will happen, because she knows she'll feel terrible if she doesn't get her workout in. She also plans her clean meals ahead of time, and before she eats anything she asks herself if that morsel will help bring her closer to or further from her goal.

MORE POSITIVES

Tammy has found that sticking to her training and eating plan gives her added bonuses. As a single working mom, she has little time to herself and finds those 30 to 60 minutes training is invaluable "me time." She also feels much better when she eats clean and her kids want to eat the same nutritious foods she does!

"Some people have been supportive and some have not," she says. "There will always be people who try to sabotage you with temptation. But the great news is no one can force you to eat something. Once you get past all that, you'll find a real shift in your mentality."

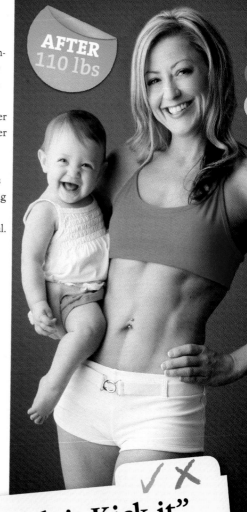

AFTER
110 lbs

"My Pick it Kick it"

BREAKFAST

PICK IT
Oatmeal with cinnamon

KICK IT
White bagels

DINNER

PICK IT
Salmon and a small yam, salad on the side

KICK IT
Pasta with alfredo sauce

MY SUCCESS TIP: "I snack on air-popped popcorn, raw veggies or rice cakes!"

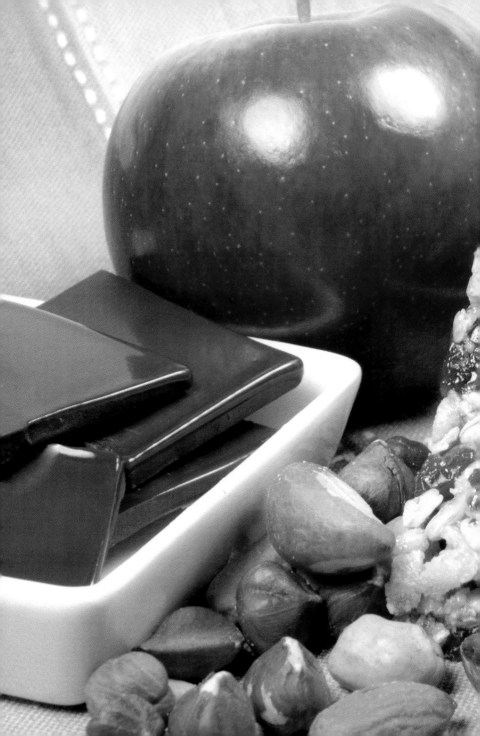

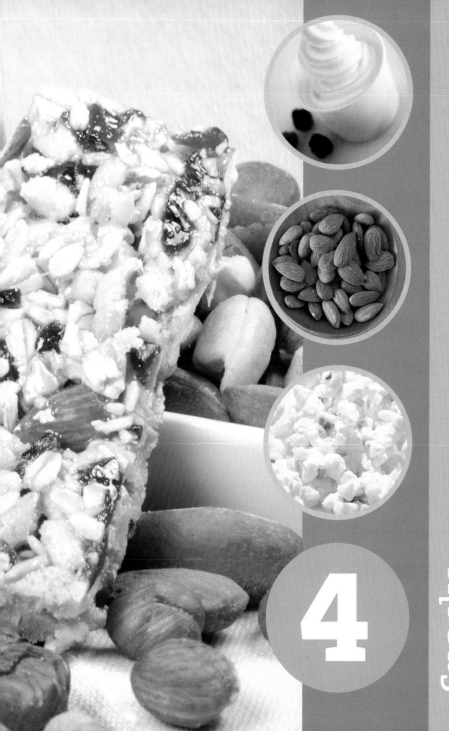

4

Snacks

GO
AHEAD,
HAVE A SNACK!

(in fact, have a few!)

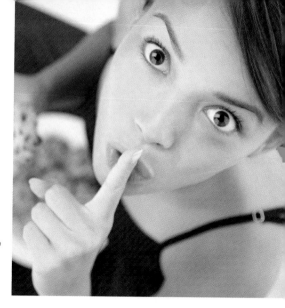

> "When I hit a mid-morning slump, I've learned to reach for an apple, some edamame, or yogurt and berries instead of a bag of chips."

I have to admit that I'm what many call a clean-eating grazer – I like to munch on something every couple of hours, be it a snack or a smaller meal.

When I hit a mid-morning slump, I've learned to reach for an apple, some edamame, or yogurt and berries instead of a bag of chips. Weaning myself off the requisite can of diet soda in the afternoon was another swap I consciously made. And you know what? I not only felt more energized, but my dentist also thanked me. Research proves soda pop and energy drinks are some of the worst offenders of tooth enamel decay.

The more you eat, the more you lose. Believe it or not, it's that simple. But it's what you choose to eat and when you eat it that makes the difference between shedding pounds and putting them on. Research shows that women snack more than twice a day [*National Health and Nutrition Examination Survey* 1999-2002] and show no signs of stopping. This can actually be a good thing – the more you snack, the better your chance of losing weight. If you don't snack, your blood sugar drops and you tend to eat more at your next meal. A small, nutrient-dense snack can keep your metabolism revving and fill you up until your next meal. So go ahead, have a snack!

In the journal *Appetite*, 2008, Barbara Rolls, PhD, author of *The Volumetrics Eating Plan* and director of the Laboratory for the Study of Human Ingestive Behavior at Penn State, served visitors either crunchy cheese snacks or puffy, aerated (full of air) snacks. The people munching the airier stuff ate nearly 75 percent more by volume but consumed fewer calories. What does this mean for you? Choose air-puffed snacks over dense ones to feel fuller on fewer calories.

PICK IT

Nutritional Value

SERVING	11 crackers
CALORIES	110
FAT	0 g
CARBS	22 g
FIBER	0.5 g
SUGAR	3 g
SODIUM	230 mg
PROTEIN	2 g

 FAST FACT

Most nutritionists recommend that healthy adults not exceed the range of 1,500 to 2,400 milligrams (mg) of sodium a day.

30

Percentage of all calories consumed by Americans from sweets, desserts, soft drinks, alcoholic beverages, salty snacks and fruit-flavored drinks. Healthy fruits and vegetables make up only 10 percent of calories consumed in the average U.S. diet.

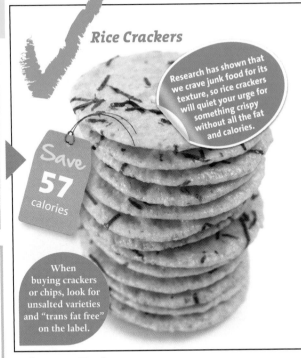

Rice Crackers

Research has shown that we crave junk food for its texture, so rice crackers will quiet your urge for something crispy without all the fat and calories.

Save **57** calories

When buying crackers or chips, look for unsalted varieties and "trans fat free" on the label.

Give It a Try!

Nabisco Garden Harvest Toasted Chips – vegetable medley
120 calories, 3.5 g fat, 240 mg sodium

True North almond crisps
140 calories, 7 g fat, 240 mg sodium

Robert's American Gourmet Rich soy crisps
120 calories, 4 g fat, 210 mg sodium

 YES YOU CAN

Eat healthy fats! Go for olive oil, peanut oil, avocados, nuts and seeds to get in nutritious monounsaturated fats. Vegetable oils (such as safflower, corn, sunflower, soy and grapeseed oils) are also good sources of healthy fats. Salmon, mackerel, herring, flaxseeds and walnuts are excellent sources of omega-3 fatty acids.

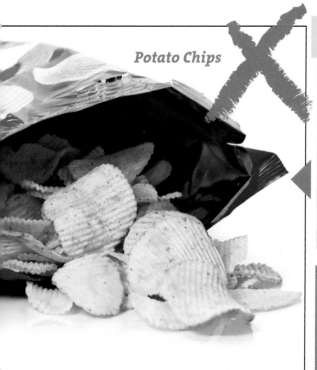

Potato Chips

KICK IT

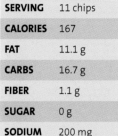

Nutritional Value	
SERVING	11 chips
CALORIES	167
FAT	11.1 g
CARBS	16.7 g
FIBER	1.1 g
SUGAR	0 g
SODIUM	200 mg
PROTEIN	2.2 g

EXCUSE
BUSTED

Think you can't avoid trans fat, the worst fat for the heart, blood vessels and rest of the body?

You might not be able to cut out trans fat completely, but small changes in your diet can make a big difference. Choose liquid vegetable oils or choose a soft tub margarine that contains little or no trans fats. Avoid eating commercially prepared baked foods (cookies, pies, donuts, etc.), snack foods and processed foods, including fast foods.

Ditch These Too!

Nabisco Ritz Toasted – sour cream and onion
130 calories, 6 g fat, 270 mg sodium

Stacy's pita chips – parmesan garlic and herb
140 calories, 5 g fat, 200 mg sodium

Goldfish baked snack crackers
160 calories, 6 g fat, 290 mg sodium

TIP To eat well, reach for plants. Load up on vegetables, fruits, whole grains and healthy fats such as olive and canola oil.

Try This
Cut down on your sodium intake. The lower the amount of sodium in your diet, the better it is for your blood pressure. Excess sodium can lead to kidney and cardiovascular diseases.

PICK IT

Nutritional Value

SERVING	1 small
CALORIES	225
FAT	11 g
CARBS	26 g
FIBER	3 g
SUGAR	0 g
SODIUM	150 mg
PROTEIN	5 g

A BETTER CHOICE

Opt for popcorn without butter to avoid consuming trans fat.

▶ QUICK & EASY

Pair your popcorn with water, coffee or tea at the movies. "Diet" drinks with artificial sweeteners may make us crave super sugary foods. Water is the best calorie-free beverage around. If it's too bland, try adding a squeeze of lemon or lime. Plain coffee and tea are also good calorie-free choices, as long as they're consumed in moderation!

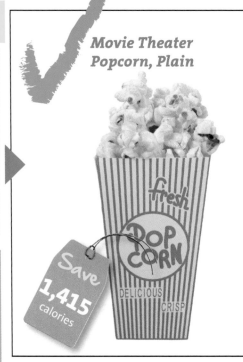

Movie Theater Popcorn, Plain

Save **1,415** calories

Give It a Try!

Planters trail mix (28 g)
150 calories, 11 g fat, 6 g sugar

Eden Organic dried cranberries (1/3 cup)
140 calories, 0.5 fat, 25 g sugar

Lindt Excellence 85% cocoa extra dark chocolate
210 calories, 18 g fat, 5 g sugar

Say What?

LOSING THOSE POUNDS will save you money in the long run. According to the National Center for Chronic Disease Prevention and Health Promotion, a 10 percent weight loss will reduce an overweight person's lifetime medical costs by $2,200 to $5,300.

Movie Theater Popcorn, with Butter

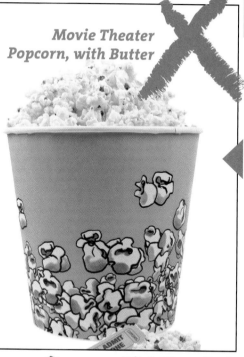

KICK IT

Nutritional Value	
SERVING	1 large
CALORIES	1,640
FAT	126 g
CARBS	94 g
FIBER	11 g
SUGAR	0 g
SODIUM	430 mg
PROTEIN	37 g

YES YOU CAN Reduce your cholesterol by making small changes in your lifestyle:

Ditch These Too!

SUGAR ALERT!

Skittles
170 calories, 2 g fat, 32 g sugar

Sour Patch Kids
140 calories, 0 fat, 25 g sugar

Snickers bar
280 calories, 14 g fat, 30 g sugar

Try This!

Feel free to splurge on popcorn once in a while, but try to cut back on other American staples. Red meat, refined grains, potatoes, sugary drinks and salty snacks are part of American culture, but not a good part. Go for a plant-based diet rich in non-starchy vegetables, fruits and whole grains. And if you eat animal protein, fish and poultry are the best choices.

- Try to shed a few pounds by looking for ways to incorporate more activity into your daily routine, such as taking the stairs instead of the elevator.

- Eat heart-healthy foods. Choose whole grain breads, whole wheat flour and brown rice. Stock up on fruits and vegetables.

- If you choose to drink, do so in moderation. This means no more than one drink a day for women, and one or two drinks a day for men. Never binge drink.

PICK IT

Nutritional Value

SERVING	1 cup
CALORIES	260
FAT	3 g
CARBS	50 g
FIBER	0 g
SUGAR	38 g
SODIUM	250 mg
PROTEIN	10 g

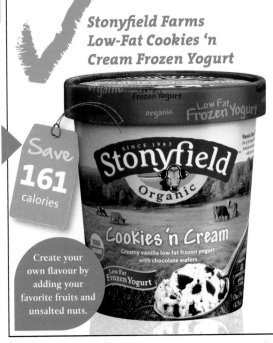

Stonyfield Farms Low-Fat Cookies 'n Cream Frozen Yogurt

Save **161** calories

Create your own flavour by adding your favorite fruits and unsalted nuts.

YES YOU CAN

Fit in two sources of calcium each day. Dairy products are best, but you can also get calcium by eating salmon with bones, sardines and dark leafy greens such as collard greens. Also, check the label: some brands of bread, tofu and orange juice are fortified with calcium.

Give It a Try!

Ben & Jerry's sorbet – berried treasure
110 calories, 0 fat, 24 g sugar

Haagen-Dazs Reserve sorbet – Brazilian açai berry
120 calories, 2 g fat, 20 g sugar

Frozen fruit bars
80 calories, 0 fat, 20 g sugar

TIP Eating a low-fat yogurt fortified with vitamin D after a workout can help decrease your body-fat percentage in just eight weeks.

Say What?

HIT THE GYM to boost your brainpower! In two new studies, Mayo Clinic researchers found that moderate exercise may reduce the risk of mild cognitive impairment associated with aging, while high-intensity aerobics may actually help those already suffering from the condition.

KICK IT

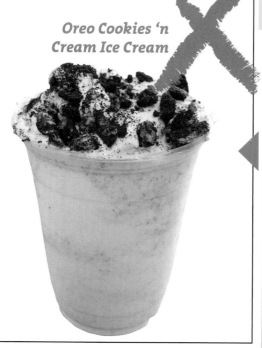

Oreo Cookies 'n Cream Ice Cream

Nutritional Value	
SERVING	1 cup
CALORIES	421
FAT	22.6 g
CARBS	48.2 g
FIBER	1.5 g
SUGAR	40.6 g
SODIUM	226 mg
PROTEIN	7.5 g

>> FAST FACT

Despite the proven benefits of physical activity, more than 60 percent of American adults do not get enough physical activity to provide health benefits.

Ditch These Too!

Nestle Drumstick – caramel
360 calories, 22 g fat, 29 g sugar

Haagen-Dazs bar – vanilla and almond
320 calories, 23 g fat, 20 g sugar

Edy's/Dreyers fruit bar – creamy coconut
120 calories, 3 g fat, 15 g sodium

BONUS!

No bones about it, you need calcium every day. Many people do not get enough of the calcium needed for strong bones and proper muscle function. Lack of calcium can contribute to stress fractures and osteoporosis. Frozen yogurt is made from dairy products, which makes it rich in calcium.

Dark Chocolate Covered Almonds

Nutritional Value	
SERVING	1 oz
CALORIES	149
FAT	12 g
CARBS	11.3 g
FIBER	2.8 g
SUGAR	7.1 g
SODIUM	21 mg
PROTEIN	3.5 g

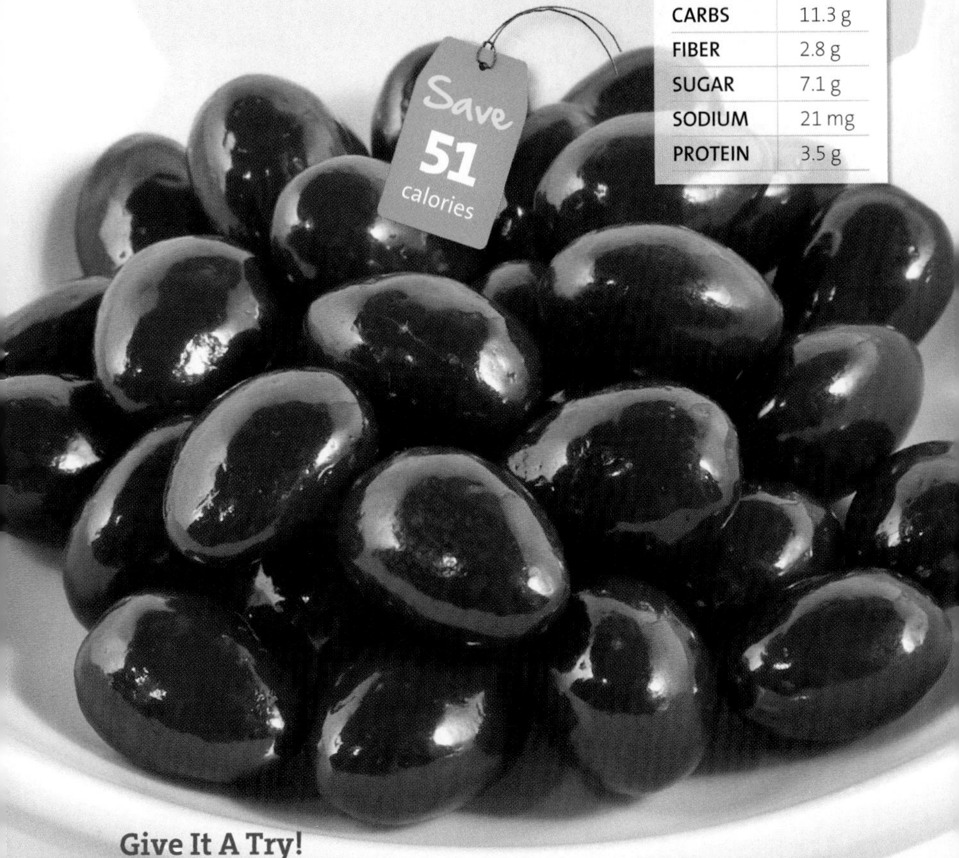

Save
51
calories

Give It A Try!

✓ **Hershey's Bliss dark chocolate (3 pieces)**
105 calories, 7 g fat, 10 g sugar

✓ **Jell-O chocolate pudding – no sugar added**
60 calories, 1 g fat, 0 g sugar

✓ **Rice Krispies Treats**
60 calories, 3 g fat, 8 g sugar

FULL OF VITAMIN E, ALMONDS ARE ALSO A BEAUTY FOOD: GREAT FOR THE HAIR AND SKIN.

SAY WHAT?
The extra calories and healthy fats are worth it! **Studies show that protein with healthy fats decreases abdominal fat.**

Try This!
Chocolate can be part of a healthy diet! Choose dark chocolate with cocoa content of 65 percent or higher. Limit yourself to no more than three ounces (85 grams) a day, which is the amount shown in studies to be helpful.

Take a deep breath and improve your health! Cutting down on stress might be difficult, but taking a moment each day to acknowledge the positive things in your life is one way to start tapping into other constructive emotions. These good feelings have been linked with better health, longer life and greater well-being, just as their opposites — chronic anger, worry, and hostility — contribute to high blood pressure and heart disease.

YES YOU CAN

KICK IT

Snack-Sized Chocolate Bars

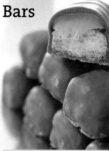

Nutritional Value

SERVING	2 "fun size" bars
CALORIES	200
FAT	8 g
CARBS	30 g
FIBER	0 g
SUGAR	20 g
SODIUM	100 mg
PROTEIN	2 g

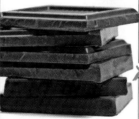

Ditch These Too!

Peanut Butter Twix
280 calories, 17 g fat, 19 g sugar

Hershey's milk chocolate
230 calories, 13 g fat, 22 g sugar

Peanut M&M's
220 calories, 11 g fat, 22 g sugar

SAY WHAT? Chocolate's main ingredient, cocoa, appears to reduce risk factors for heart disease. Cocoa beans have antioxidant effects that reduce cell damage implicated in heart disease. Cocoa also helps lower blood pressure and improve vascular function. Dark chocolate is more effective than milk chocolate at reducing risk factors for cardiovascular problems.

PICK IT

Nutritional Value

SERVING	42 g (1 bag)
CALORIES	130
FAT	0 g
CARBS	30 g
FIBER	4 g
SUGAR	24 g
SODIUM	0 mg
PROTEIN	2 g

Peeled Snacks
Cherry-Go-Round

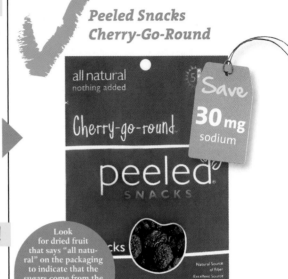

all natural
nothing added

Cherry-go-round

peeled
SNACKS

Save
30 mg
sodium

Look for dried fruit that says "all natural" on the packaging to indicate that the sugars come from the fruit and are not added in. Always check the ingredients list.

NET WT 1.48 OZ (42g)

Natural Source of Fiber
Excellent Source of Vitamin C

BONUS!

Peeled Snacks
Cherry-go-round
is a good source of
fiber and Vitamin C.

▶ QUICK & EASY

A great way to eat well
is to eat one extra fruit
or vegetable a day.
Fruits and vegetables
are inexpensive, taste
good and are good for ev-
erything from your brain
to your bowels.

Give It a Try!

Planters pistachio lovers mix
160 calories, 13 g fat, 80 mg sodium

Ocean Spray Craisins
130 calories, 0 fat, 26 g sugar

Planters mixed nuts and raisins mix
150 calories, 11 g fat, 6 g sugar

YES YOU CAN Eat well and have great skin! A healthy diet can help promote
healthy skin. In particular, foods that are rich in antioxidants seem
to have a great effect on the skin. For the best skin, choose fruits,
especially cherries, berries, melons, apples and pears, and vegetables, especially spinach and other leafy greens, eggplant, asparagus,
celery and onions.

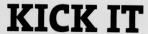

Welch's Fruit Snacks
White Grape Strawberry

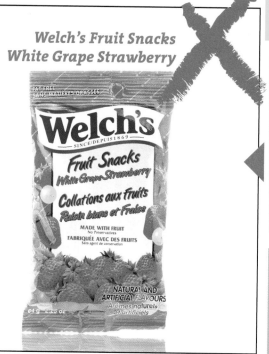

KICK IT

Nutritional Value	
SERVING	40 g (1 bag)
CALORIES	130
FAT	0 g
CARBS	31 g
FIBER	0 g
SUGAR	19 g
SODIUM	30 mg
PROTEIN	1 g

>> FAST FACT

According to Centers for Disease Control and Prevention, only about one fourth of U.S. adults eat the recommended five or more servings of fruits and vegetables each day.

Ditch These Too!
Fruit Roll-Ups – strawberry
50 calories, 1 g fat, 7 g sugar

Sun Maid yogurt cranberries
120 calories, 3.5 g fat, 20 g sugar

Planters Select macadamias, cashews and pistachios
180 calories, 17 g fat, 95 mg sodium

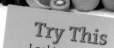

Try This
Looking for great fruits and vegetables to snack on? The Mayo Clinic lists these easily available foods as great choices: apples, blueberries, broccoli, red beans, spinach and sweet potatoes.

TIP Trying to fit exercise into a busy day but can't make it to a gym? Lifting a hardcover book or two-pound weights a few times a day can help tone your arm muscles.

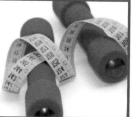

PICK IT

Nutritional Value

SERVING	1 bar
CALORIES	150
FAT	0.5 g
CARBS	35 g
FIBER	3 g
SUGAR	21 g
SODIUM	110 mg
PROTEIN	1 g

ReBar Organic Fruit & Veggie Bar

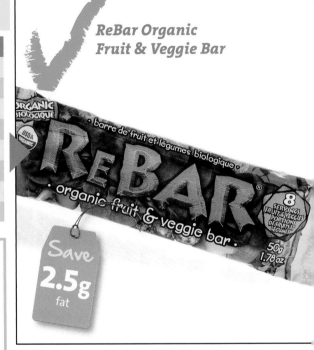

Save **2.5g** fat

▶▶ FAST FACT

Many processed foods are made with high fructose corn syrup and other sweeteners that are high in calories and low on nutrition. Regularly including these products in your diet has the potential to lead to weight gain – which, in turn, promotes conditions such as type 2 diabetes, high blood pressure and coronary artery disease.

Give It a Try!

Kashi cereal bar – ripe strawberry
110 calories, 3 g fat, 9 g sugar

Fiber One bar – oats & chocolate
140 calories, 4 g fat, 10 g sugar

Quaker Chewy bar
100 calories, 3g fat, 7 g sugar

YES YOU CAN

Eat cleaner by cutting down on high fructose corn syrup!
Follow these tips to cut down on corn syrup and other sweeteners:
- Avoid foods that contain added sugar.
- Choose fresh fruit rather than fruit juice or fruit-flavored drinks. Even 100 percent fruit juice has a high concentration of sugar.
- Choose fruit canned in its own juices instead of heavy syrup.
- Drink less soda.
- Don't allow sweetened beverages to replace milk or water, especially for children.

Nutri-Grain Bars

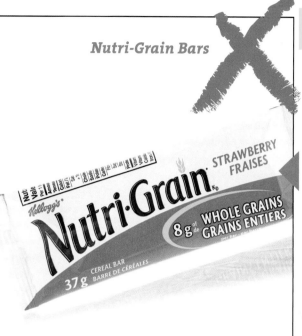

Nutritional Value	
SERVING	1 bar
CALORIES	140
FAT	3 g
CARBS	26 g
FIBER	1 g
SUGAR	13 g
SODIUM	110 mg
PROTEIN	1 g

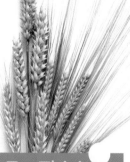

Ditch These Too!

Hostess breakfast bar – banana nut
130 calories, 2.5 g fat, 17 g sugar

Kashi Go Lean bar – cookies 'n cream
290 calories, 6 g fat, 35 g sugar

Kudos granola bar – peanut butter
130 calories, 6 g fat, 10 g sugar

FATTER, NOT FITTER

Tempted to reach for a Nutri-Grain bar as part of a healthy diet? Items such as these may sound healthy, but they're not! Nutri-Grain bars are made with some whole grains, but the second ingredient is enriched flour. What's more, these bars contain high fructose corn syrup.

Try This!

Look for whole grain stamps on food packages at your grocery store: they help consumers identify foods made with whole grains. It's recommended that you aim for at least 48 grams of whole grains each day. Eating just three servings of products labeled "100% Whole Grain" will get you your whole grain fill for the day. If the label just says "Whole Grain" you'll need to eat six servings to get your daily dose.

PICK IT

Nutritional Value

SERVING	10 nuts
CALORIES	39
FAT	3.1 g
CARBS	2 g
FIBER	0.7 g
SUGAR	0.5 g
SODIUM	0.1 mg
PROTEIN	1.4 g

Pistachios

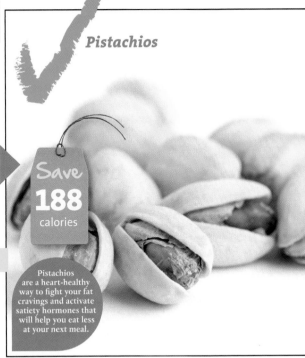

Save
188
calories

Pistachios are a heart-healthy way to fight your fat cravings and activate satiety hormones that will help you eat less at your next meal.

BONUS!

Unsalted

pistachios contain high amounts of potassium and low amounts of sodium which helps to regulate blood pressure, stabilize water balance in the body and strengthen muscles. Pistachios are also a good source of vitamin E, which boosts the immune system and alleviates fatigue.

Give It a Try!

Sunsweet California pitted dates
120 calories, 0 fat, 0 sodium

Planters pecan lovers mix
180 calories, 17 g fat, 70 mg sodium

Blue Diamond whole natural almonds
170 calories, 14 g fat, 0 sodium

Say What?

HEALTHY ADULTS NEED no more than 2,400 milligrams of sodium per day. This is the amount of sodium in one teaspoon of salt.

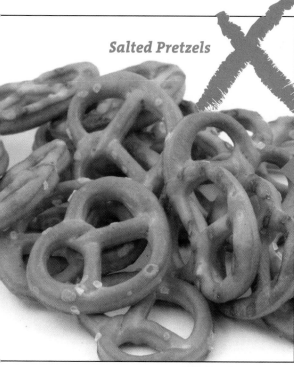

Salted Pretzels

KICK IT

>> **FAST FACT**

Women increased their daily calorie consumption 22 percent between 1971 and 2000, from 1,542 calories per day to 1,877 calories. The calorie intake for men increased seven percent from 2,450 calories per day to 2,618 calories.

Ditch These Too!

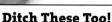

Planters dry roasted peanuts, salted
170 calories, 14 g fat, 190 mg sodium

Planters nut and chocolate trail mix
160 calories, 10 g fat, 25 mg sodium

Diamond chopped pecans
210 calories, 22 g fat, 0 sodium

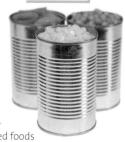

>> **HOW DO YOU CUT BACK ON SODIUM?** The good news is you can cut down on sodium by simply switching from processed foods to fresh foods. You can also look for the low-sodium versions of packaged food.

- Choose fresh or frozen vegetables instead of canned.
- Choose low-sodium broth and soups.
- Limit cured meats or foods packed in brine; choose fresh meats instead.
- Limit instant foods such as instant rice, noodles and frozen dinners.
- Rinse and drain canned foods such as canned beans, if possible.

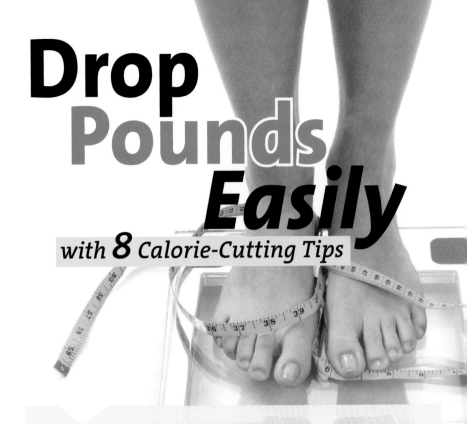

Drop Pounds *Easily*

with *8* Calorie-Cutting Tips

To lose ten pounds in five to eight weeks, you'll need to cut about 200 calories a day. And to lose 15 pounds in 8 to 12 weeks, cut 300 to 350 calories a day. How do you do that? Use these easy calorie-cutting tips!

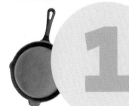

1

When sautéing veggies and meat, substitute a couple of quick sprays of PAM for oil or butter. You'll save 100 calories.

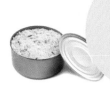

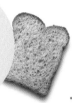

2 Choose low-sodium tuna packed in water rather than oil and save 70 calories per three ounces.

3 Slice 120 calories off your lunch by having an open-faced sandwich.

4 Instead of a serving of raisins, go for a serving of grapes to save 65 calories per ounce.

5 Roll off 100 to 140 calories by turning a wrap into a salad.

6 In shakes, sandwiches or by the spoonful, peanut and almond butters can be energy dense. Save 94 calories by using one rather than two tablespoons per serving.

7 Downsize meat portions by one ounce and you'll shave off 50 calories.

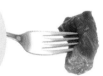

8 High fiber whole grain foods are great for staving off cravings, but go for sprouted grain products and you'll save even more calories.

PICK IT

Nutritional Value

SERVING	1 orange
CALORIES	62
FAT	0.1 g
CARBS	15.5 g
FIBER	3.1 g
SUGAR	12.2 g
SODIUM	0 mg
PROTEIN	1.2 g

A BETTER CHOICE

Stop drinking your calories! You can consume a lot of calories and sugar by drinking sugar-sweetened beverages such as SunnyD and cola. Toss them in favor of water, herbal tea and decaffeinated coffee.

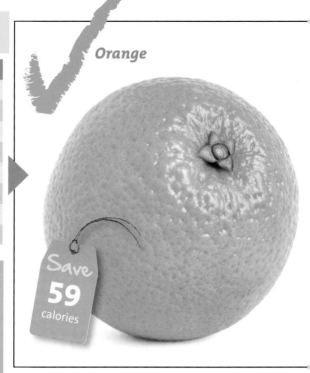

Orange

Save **59** calories

Give It a Try!

Apple
77 calories, 0.3 g fat, 15.5 g sugar

Grapes (1 cup)
62 calories, 0.4 g fat, 15 g sugar

Pomegranate (½ cup arils)
72 calories, 1 g fat, 11.9 g sugar

Say What?

ORANGE JUICE has plenty of vitamin C, but the nutritional problem with juice of any kind is that it is extracted from the fruit pulp, which contains most of the fiber and the minerals (calcium, for example) and vitamins (like beta-carotene) that go with it. Overall, whole fruits are a better nutritional bet than juices, and fresh juices are better than frozen.

Pulp-Free Orange Juice

KICK IT

Nutritional Value	
SERVING	1 cup
CALORIES	121
FAT	0.5 g
CARBS	28 g
FIBER	0.5 g
SUGAR	22.6 g
SODIUM	3 mg
PROTEIN	1.9 g

≫ FAST FACT

In Food Rules: An Eater's Manual, *Michael Pollan argues that individuals who rely on the so-called Western diet – lots of processed foods, meat, added fat, sugar and refined grains – "invariably suffer from high rates of the so-called Western diseases: obesity, type 2 diabetes, cardiovascular disease and cancer."*

Ditch These Too!

Apple juice box
100 calories, 0 fat, 22 g sugar

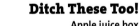

Grape juice (1 cup)
160 calories, 0 fat, 37 g sugar

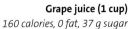

Pomegranate blueberry juice
140 calories, 0 fat, 34 g sugar

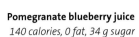

Try This

When you see a juice labelled "pulp free," this means most of the nutrients have been removed from it. Look for another option.

YES YOU CAN

Leave the sports drinks for athletes! Sports beverages are designed to give athletes simple carbs, electrolytes and fluid during high-intensity workouts that last an hour or more. If your workouts aren't that intense, these drinks are just another source of sugary calories.

PICK IT

Nutritional Value

SERVING	28 chips
CALORIES	130
FAT	7 g
CARBS	15 g
FIBER	1 g
SUGAR	1 g
SODIUM	250 mg
PROTEIN	1 g

▶ QUICK & EASY

Keep several bags of your favorite frozen vegetables on hand. Mix any combination, microwave and top with your favorite low-fat dressing. Enjoy three to four cups a day for a great snack or alternative to a salad.

MAKE IT BETTER

Eat more colors! According to Swedish researchers, the greater the variety of colors of vegetables you eat, the more antioxidants you consume to fight chronic diseases and cancers, including ovarian cancer.

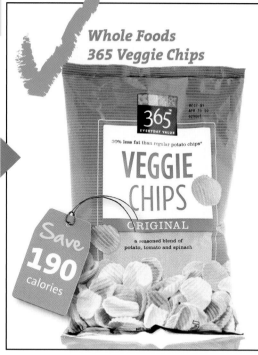

Whole Foods 365 Veggie Chips

365 EVERYDAY VALUE

30% less fat than regular potato chips*

VEGGIE CHIPS

ORIGINAL

a seasoned blend of potato, tomato and spinach

Save **190** calories

Give It a Try!

Kettle Bakes – lightly salted
120 calories, 3 g fat, 115 mg sodium

Pringles Minis – sour cream and onion
130 calories, 8 g fat, 170 mg sodium

Terra Blues chips
130 calories, 6 g fat, 115 mg sodium

YES YOU CAN Fit in a quick workout during your workday. Squeeze a run in during lunch if you're not a morning person. Bring your workout clothes, run around the block at lunch and be back at work ready to tackle the afternoon.

Pringles Chips, Original

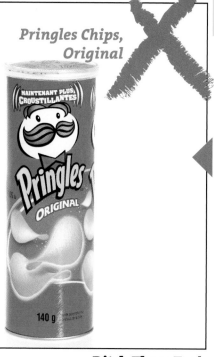

EXCUSE
BUSTED

I'm bored with my exercise routine.

Change it up. Sure, walking or running every day can be fun and effective. But throwing some swimming, biking, strength workouts or kickboxing into the mix can alleviate boredom, help prevent injury and you get into better shape. Try a different aerobics class at your gym or give yoga or pilates a go.

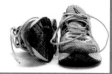
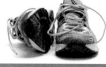

Ditch These Too!

Ruffles – cheddar and sour cream
160 calories, 11 g fat, 230 mg

Lay's – sour cream and onion
160 calories, 10 g fat, 210 mg sodium

Lay's – dill pickle
140 calories, 10 g fat, 150 mg sodium

TIP Instead of whole milk, switch to one percent. If you drink one glass a day, you'll lose five pounds in a year!

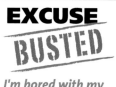

PICK IT

Nutritional Value

SERVING	12 fl oz
CALORIES	318
FAT	8.4 g
CARBS	51.6 g
FIBER	0 g
SUGAR	41.4 g
SODIUM	156 mg
PROTEIN	8.4 g

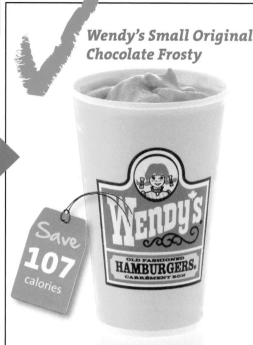

Wendy's Small Original Chocolate Frosty

Save **107** calories

EXCUSE BUSTED

I can't get motivated to work out anymore.

Feeling sluggish? Signing up for a 5K or a triathlon are my favorite motivators. Knowing I have a race coming up inspires me to get to the gym and train hard because otherwise I might be lapped by faster athletes. Competing is a fun way to push yourself to reach your fitness goals.

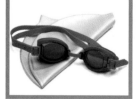

Give It a Try!
Medium iced tea
142 calories, 0 fat, 36 g sugar

Wendy's small hot cocoa
120 calories, 2 g fat, 16 g sugar

Mandarin orange cup
80 calories, 0 fat, 17 g sugar

A BETTER CHOICE

When dining out, make it automatic: order one dessert to share. Split the Wendy's Frosty with a friend and cut your dessert calories in half.

McDonald's Chocolate Triple Thick Shake (12 oz)

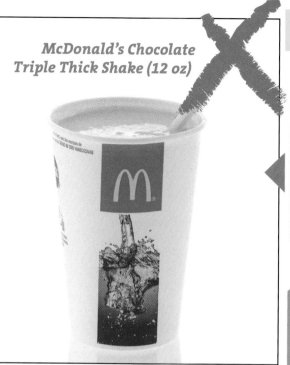

KICK IT

Nutritional Value	
SERVING	12 fl oz
CALORIES	425
FAT	10.1 g
CARBS	76.1 g
FIBER	0.8 g
SUGAR	63 g
SODIUM	191 mg
PROTEIN	10.1 g

ALL YOU!

Be conscious about what you put in your mouth—don't allow yourself to graze on bad choices. You can easily munch away hundreds of calories of cereal or chips without realizing it.

Ditch These Too!

McDonald's Cinnamon Melts
460 calories, 19 g fat, 32 g sugar

Iced coffee – caramel (regular)
190 calories, 8 g fat, 27.8 g sugar

McDonald's Apple Pie
270 calories, 12 g fat, 13 g sugar

TIP Enjoy eating and engage with your food. Make eating purposeful, not absentminded. Whenever you put food in your mouth, chew it slowly and savor it. Engage all of your senses whether indulging in a snack or eating a meal.

Try This

Fill up on the good stuff first. Eat the low-calorie items on your plate first and then move on to fattier options. Start with salads, veggies and broth-based soups, and eat meats and starches last. By the time you get to them, you'll be full enough to be satisfied with smaller portions.

Cherry Jell-O

Save 550 calories

Nutritional Value

SERVING	1 package
CALORIES	80
FAT	0 g
CARBS	20 g
FIBER	0 g
SUGAR	19 g
SODIUM	40 mg
PROTEIN	1 g

Cube cold Jell-O and mix with fruit for a delicious snack.

Give It A Try!

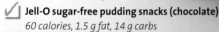 **Jell-O sugar-free pudding snacks (chocolate)**
60 calories, 1.5 g fat, 14 g carbs

Mott's organic unsweetened applesauce cups
50 calories, 0 fat, 12 g carbs

Yoplait fat-free yogurt – key lime pie
100 calories, 0 fat, 17 g carbs

FATTER, NOT FITTER

- **Check that label!** Don't assume that all energy bars and fruit smoothies are low in calories and fat.

Nutrition Facts
Amount Per Serving
Calories 200 Calories from Fat 90

	% Daily Value*
Total Fat 10g	**15%**
Saturated Fat 5g	25%
Trans Fat 0g	
Cholesterol 0mg	**0%**
Sodium 100mg	**4%**

YES YOU CAN

Stay motivated with your fitness goals. Get some good gear to work out in. If you reach a goal, give yourself a reward — an mp3 player, a heart rate monitor or pedometer. Having great gear can make you look forward to your workouts.

EXCUSE BUSTED

I feel tired during my workouts. Make sure you fuel up. If your workout will be more than 30 minutes long, you really should have some energy in you before starting. Eat a banana or some toast with peanut butter an hour before your workout, and you'll find yourself with more energy to reach your fitness goals.

ALL THE CHERRY FLAVOR, FOR A FRACTION OF THE SUGAR CONTENT.

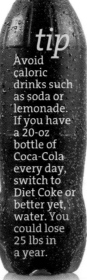

tip

Avoid caloric drinks such as soda or lemonade. If you have a 20-oz bottle of Coca-Cola every day, switch to Diet Coke or better yet, water. You could lose 25 lbs in a year.

SAY WHAT? You may not know that eating foods made with gelatin, such as Jell-O, has health benefits. Gelatin promotes a feeling of fullness, maintains regularity, and helps to strengthen hair and nails. It also appears to be beneficial to athletes for muscle growth and metabolism.

KICK IT

Cherry Cheesecake

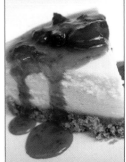

Nutritional Value

SERVING	1 slice
CALORIES	630
FAT	45 g
CARBS	53 g
FIBER	0 g
SUGAR	42 g
SODIUM	390 mg
PROTEIN	12 g

Ditch These Too!

Jell-O pudding snacks (chocolate)
140 calories, 4 g fat, 27 g carbs

Mott's classic applesauce cups
100 calories, 0 fat, 24 g carbs

Yoplait Thick & Creamy yogurt – key kime pie
190 calories, 3.5 g fat, 32 g carbs

PICK IT

Nutritional Value	
SERVING	9 mini cakes
CALORIES	70
FAT	2.5 g
CARBS	11 g
FIBER	0 g
SUGAR	1 g
SODIUM	200 mg
PROTEIN	1 g

A BETTER CHOICE

Eating out? Ask the server to bag half of your meal. A typical restaurant entree has 1,000 to 2,000 calories, not even counting the bread, drink and dessert!

Try This

Start a blog! Record your diet, exercise and weight goals, and share them with friends. Positive public pressure can be motivating. Commit to one exercise or nutrition goal per month and post your results every week.

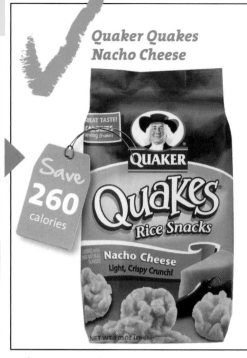

Quaker Quakes Nacho Cheese

Save **260** calories

QUAKER
Quakes
Rice Snacks
Nacho Cheese
Light, Crispy Crunch!
NET WT 3.03 OZ (86 g)

Give It a Try!

Baked Doritos – nacho cheese
120 calories, 3.5 g fat, 220 mg sodium

Sun Chips
140 calories, 6 g fat, 120 mg sodium

Guiltless Gourmet – chili lime
120 calories, 3 g fat, 250 mg sodium

YES YOU CAN

Defeat your sugar habit. The average can of sugary soda or fruit punch contains about 150 calories of pure sugar. Cut back on sugar-sweetened drinks to control your weight and to help lower your risk of developing type 2 diabetes.

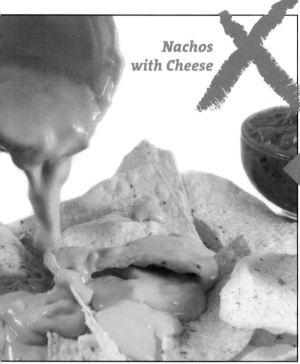

Nachos with Cheese

KICK IT

Nutritional Value	
SERVING	1 small serving
CALORIES	330
FAT	21 g
CARBS	32 g
FIBER	2 g
SUGAR	3 g
SODIUM	530 mg
PROTEIN	4 g

EXCUSE BUSTED

I don't eat veggies.

Try to eat just one or two fruit or veggie servings daily. Get comfortable with that goal and then add one extra serving at a time until you reach eight to ten a day. A great way of getting in those veggies is to make sure your plate is half veggies and/or fruit at both lunch and dinner.

Ditch These Too!

Fritos
160 calories, 10 g fat, 160 mg sodium

Tostitos – hint of lime
150 calories, 8 g fat, 160 mg sodium

Doritos – smokin' barbeque cheddar
150 calories, 8 g fat, 180 sodium

Say What?

LOOK FOR CALCIUM beyond the dairy aisle. Non-dairy foods rich in calcium include leafy green vegetables and broccoli, both of which are also great sources of vitamin K, another nutrient for strong bones.

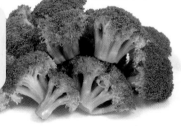

PICK IT

Nutritional Value	
SERVING	1 cake
CALORIES	60
FAT	1 g
CARBS	12 g
FIBER	0 g
SUGAR	4 g
SODIUM	35 mg
PROTEIN	1 g

Say What?

DON'T OVERDO IT! If you have a hard workout today, take it easy tomorrow. Don't work out intensely two days in a row, or you risk overtraining and injury. The hard/easy approach is also beneficial within a single workout. Go hard, then easy, and then hard again. Mixing up tempos helps you burn more fat than if you just keep a steady pace the whole time.

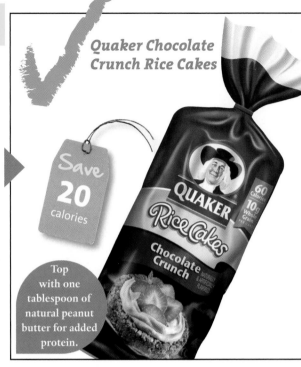

Quaker Chocolate Crunch Rice Cakes

Save **20** calories

Top with one tablespoon of natural peanut butter for added protein.

Give It a Try!
Fat-Free Fig Newtons (2 cookies)
90 calories, 0 fat, 12 g sugar

Rice Krispies Treats
90 calories, 2.5 g fat, 7 g sugar

Almond biscotti (1 cookie)
70 calories, 3.2 g fat, 4.2 g sugar

≫ *FAST FACT*

Stick to one type of cookie or flavor of ice cream. Seeing too many options can lead you to underestimate serving sizes and overeat. – Journal of Consumer Research

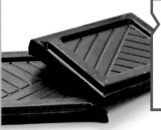

TIP Chocolate craving? Stick to dark varieties – the higher the cocoa percentage, the more antioxidants and the less sugar.

KICK IT

Chips Ahoy Chunky Chocolate Cookies

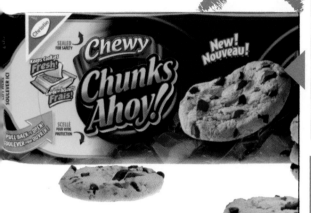

Nutritional Value	
SERVING	1 cookie
CALORIES	80
FAT	4 g
CARBS	10 g
FIBER	1 g
SUGAR	6 g
SODIUM	55 mg
PROTEIN	1 g

EXCUSE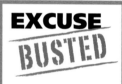

Find yourself famished and there's only a vending machine in sight?

If you have no alternative but an office vending machine, reach for the nuts – they offer more nutrition than anything else available.

Ditch These Too!

Josephine's date & nut cookies (2 cookies)
280 calories, 12 g fat, 22 g sugar

Double Stuf Oreos
140 calories, 7 g fat, 20 g sugar

Shortbread (1 cookie)
90 calories, 5 g fat, 3 g sugar

❯ QUICK & EASY

Craving something sweet? You can have about 150 calories per day of your favorite treat without sidetracking your nutrition goals. One ounce of chocolate, half a modest slice of cake, or a half-cup of ice cream once a day is okay, as long as you stick to one serving only!

TIP Have a glass or two of V8 or tomato juice instead of a Diet Coke in the mid-afternoon.

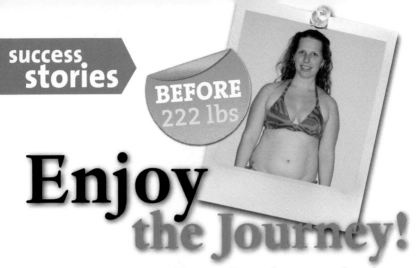

BEFORE
222 lbs

Enjoy
the Journey!

After allowing herself to eat lots of processed carbs, sweets and fatty foods during her pregnancy, this formerly fit gal had to face lots of extra fat once her baby was born! BY WENDY MORLEY

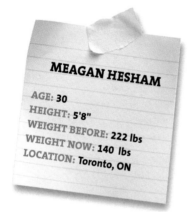

MEAGAN HESHAM

AGE: 30
HEIGHT: 5'8"
WEIGHT BEFORE: 222 lbs
WEIGHT NOW: 140 lbs
LOCATION: Toronto, ON

Meagan makes a point of staying positive, believing in herself and rewarding herself when she reaches her goals.

A dance instructor and owner of her own dance studio, Meagan had always eaten quite well and stayed in shape. She worked out, walked a lot and continued teaching dance right up until her baby was born, so she didn't gain weight from lack of exercise. Nope, it was her diet. "I let myself eat anything I wanted," she says. "I knew it wasn't right and that I was gaining way too much weight, but it was so easy because everyone blamed it on my pregnancy."

PICTURES DON'T LIE!
While she knew she had some extra fat, as is the case with many people, Meagan didn't realize just how much weight she'd gained until she had someone take some front, side and rear pictures of her in a bikini. That was a big eye opener for her and it motivated her to get back to her old fit self.

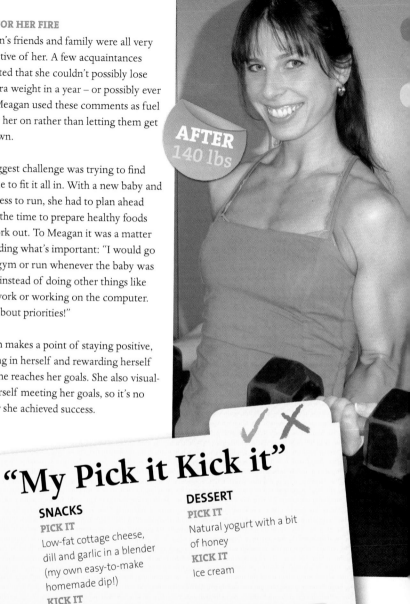

FUEL FOR HER FIRE

Meagan's friends and family were all very supportive of her. A few acquaintances suggested that she couldn't possibly lose the extra weight in a year – or possibly ever – but Meagan used these comments as fuel to spur her on rather than letting them get her down.

Her biggest challenge was trying to find the time to fit it all in. With a new baby and a business to run, she had to plan ahead to find the time to prepare healthy foods and work out. To Meagan it was a matter of deciding what's important: "I would go to the gym or run whenever the baby was asleep, instead of doing other things like housework or working on the computer. It's all about priorities!"

Meagan makes a point of staying positive, believing in herself and rewarding herself when she reaches her goals. She also visualized herself meeting her goals, so it's no wonder she achieved success.

AFTER
140 lbs

"My Pick it Kick it"

SNACKS

PICK IT
Low-fat cottage cheese, dill and garlic in a blender (my own easy-to-make homemade dip!)

KICK IT
High-fat creamy dips

DESSERT

PICK IT
Natural yogurt with a bit of honey

KICK IT
Ice cream

MY SUCCESS TIP: "One small change that's made a difference is substituting a small whole wheat tortilla to make wraps instead of using breads for sandwiches."

Menu

5

Eating Out

●●⑤ Eating Out

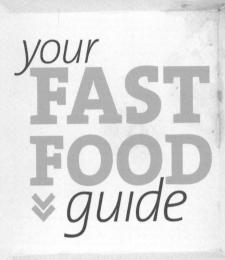

your **FAST FOOD** *guide*

Grabbing a bite doesn't have to mean packing on the pounds. Make the right swaps and shed some fat!

I have to admit, I simply love to go out to dinner. To take time to savor a meal that someone else cooks and, even better, serves, is a treat I'll never tire of. And it seems I am not alone. Even in this economic climate, Americans continue to eat out – we might choose to downscale our choices and, as growing numbers prove, forgo appetizers and desserts, but we still enjoy the ritual of eating away from home.

Eating out makes it easy to overindulge. One glass of wine too many, one extra appetizer and one larger-than-average portion of salad dressing means one evening can set your weight loss efforts back a week. Imagine this: butter on your bread, creamy pasta sauce and calorie-laden dessert can mean a whopping 2,000 calories, not to mention the extra sodium and fat! But with more and more restaurants catering to the healthy demands of consumers like you and me, eating out doesn't have to be a gorge-fest. In fact, if you choose wisely you can even stay on the healthy eating track, plus enjoy having someone else serve you and clean up!

ALL YOU NEED IS A LITTLE PLANNING.

Just like impulse shopping, when it comes to going out to your favorite restaurant, you have to be mindful. Take a moment to plan ahead and make a pact with yourself to not give in to the urge of a side of fries or large piece of chocolate cake. You know what I do? I actually write it down. Before I go out, I have a ritual – I pour myself a big glass of water with a slice of lemon and make a list of what I may choose. Sometimes, like 89 percent of today's consumers, I go online to look at the menu. That way, there are no surprises – I know exactly what choices I have and how best to order them, without any temptations getting in the way. Hello, grilled shrimp and salad with dressing on the side, and welcome, looser-fitting clothes!

CAN YOU EAT WHATEVER YOU WANT
IF YOU BURN IT OFF?

Leafing through *The Diet Detective's Countdown* (Fireside, 2007) you might think so. Author Charles Stuart Platkin, MPH, categorizes food and how many minutes of exercise is equal to the caloric value of specific foods. "There is a danger if you think you have to swim off everything that you eat," warns Platkin.

Beware though: Just because something is low-calorie doesn't mean that it's healthy for you. Look for good sources of nutrients.

Check This Out!

FOOD	CALORIES	WALK	RUN	SWIM
½ cup frozen yogurt	110	28 MIN	12 MIN	13 MIN
½ cup sugar-free frozen yogurt	100	26 MIN	11 MIN	12 MIN
½ cup rainbow sherbet	130	34 MIN	14 MIN	16 MIN
1 slice cheesecake	257	66 MIN	27 MIN	31 MIN
1 slice coconut custard pie	390	101 MIN	42 MIN	47 MIN

Eating Out At ARBY'S

PICK IT ✓   KICK IT ✗

Regular Roast Beef Sandwich			Roast Beef & Swiss Sandwich		
	SERVING	1 sandwich		SERVING	1 sandwich
	CALORIES	350		CALORIES	820
	FAT	13 g		FAT	37 g
	CARBS	37 g		CARBS	84 g
Try it without the sauce!	FIBER	2 g		FIBER	6 g
	SUGAR	5 g		SUGAR	18 g
Save 800 mg sodium	SODIUM	960 mg		SODIUM	1,760 mg
	PROTEIN	23 g		PROTEIN	40 g

Chopped Farmhouse Chicken Salad (Roasted or Grilled) with Balsamic Vinaigrette Dressing			Chopped Farmhouse Chicken Salad (Crispy) with Butter- milk Ranch Dressing		
	SERVING	1 salad		SERVING	1 salad
	CALORIES	390		CALORIES	660
	FAT	26 g		FAT	48 g
	CARBS	15 g		CARBS	31 g
Save 270 calories	FIBER	3 g		FIBER	4 g
	SUGAR	10 g		SUGAR	6 g
	SODIUM	1,240 mg		SODIUM	1,470 mg
	PROTEIN	26 g		PROTEIN	33 g

TIP Get in that iron

Pre-menopausal women simply need more iron to replace what they lose during their monthly cycles. Iron-deficiency anemia is also very common in young women. Regularly include iron-rich foods such as meat, shellfish, beans and enriched cereals in your diet to ensure that you don't become iron deficient.

Say What?

SINCE THE 1970s, portion sizes in restaurants have increased up to five times. Between 1970 and 1996, according to a report from the USDA, added fats and oils in the food supply chain have shot up a whopping 22 percent.

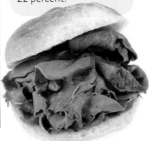

YES YOU CAN

Pamper yourself and keep on track with your fitness and nutrition goals! Come up with a self-care menu and order up one item each day to reward yourself and boost your energy. Some menu items could include: meditation, meeting up for iced tea with friends, going to bed early, dancing to at least one song in your house every day or saying "no" to one time commitment.

PICK IT ✓   KICK IT ✗

Grilled Chicken Sandwich				Chicken Salad Sandwich		
SERVING	1 order			SERVING	1 order
CALORIES	441			CALORIES	637
FAT	19 g			FAT	37 g
CARBS	33 g			CARBS	54 g
FIBER	2 g			FIBER	6 g
SUGAR	4 g			SUGAR	11 g
SODIUM	971 mg			SODIUM	1,293 mg
PROTEIN	35 g			PROTEIN	22 g

Save 322 mg sodium

Grilled Cheese Sandwich				Bob's BLT & E		
SERVING	1 order			SERVING	1 order
CALORIES	350			CALORIES	639
FAT	15 g			FAT	41 g
CARBS	22 g			CARBS	26 g
FIBER	2 g			FIBER	3 g
SUGAR	4 g			SUGAR	6 g
SODIUM	729 mg			SODIUM	1,021 mg
PROTEIN	9 g			PROTEIN	19 g

Save 289 calories

ALL YOU!

Make sure you're not taking too many supplements. Vitamin pills are meant to complement your diet, not act as a stand-in for the foods you don't eat. Taking too many vitamins can end up sabotaging your good health. Experts recommend taking no more than one all-purpose multivitamin daily.

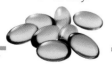

YES YOU CAN

Get in a great workout by creating a simple but challenging fitness program. Make sure your regular routine includes the multi-purpose squat, which strengthens all of the major muscles of the lower body, including the gluteals, hamstrings, quadriceps and calves. Other top exercise choices include running, abdominal exercises, lunges, walking, push-ups and yoga.

Say What?

NUTRITION ISN'T ALL ABOUT WHAT YOU EAT.
While most folks believe nutrition is all about food, it's also about how your body uses food and that's where regular exercise comes in. Without regular exercise, you cannot maintain a high enough metabolic rate to burn your food efficiently.

PICK IT ✓

KICK IT ✗

Whopper Jr. Sandwich

Hold the mayo and save more sodium and fat!

SERVING	1 order
CALORIES	370
FAT	21 g
CARBS	31 g
FIBER	2 g
SUGAR	6 g
SODIUM	560 mg
PROTEIN	16 g

Save 460 mg sodium

Whopper Sandwich

SERVING	1 order
CALORIES	670
FAT	40 g
CARBS	51 g
FIBER	3 g
SUGAR	11 g
SODIUM	1,020 mg
PROTEIN	29 g

Hamburger

Hold the ketchup and save even more sodium!

SERVING	1 order
CALORIES	290
FAT	12 g
CARBS	30 g
FIBER	1 g
SUGAR	6 g
SODIUM	550 mg
PROTEIN	15 g

Save 660 calories

Steakhouse Burger

SERVING	1 order
CALORIES	950
FAT	59 g
CARBS	55 g
FIBER	4 g
SUGAR	12 g
SODIUM	1,950 mg
PROTEIN	40 g

35

Percentage of American total food spending shelled out on take-out foods in 1999. This is an increase from 25 percent in 1970.

MAKE IT BETTER

Don't be afraid to order "kid's size" burgers and meals! They can fill you up and save you a ton of calories, fat and sodium!

TIP Eat breakfast to lose weight! When it comes to cutting calories, breakfast is often the first thing to go. But new research suggests that people who are successful at losing weight — and keeping it off — eat breakfast every day. Researchers believe that eating breakfast helps people control both their hunger and food intake throughout the day.

Say What?

BUILD STRONGER muscles for a stronger brain! An active lifestyle has benefits beyond a fit body. A new study suggests that being active can stimulate brain cell growth and lower the risk of developing Alzheimer's disease.

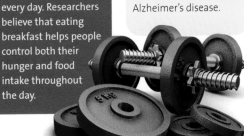

PICK IT ✓ KICK IT ✗

Big Hamburger	SERVING	1 order		Western Bacon Six Dollar Burger	SERVING	1 order
	CALORIES	460			CALORIES	1,020
	FAT	17 g			FAT	53 g
	CARBS	54 g	Save **560** calories		CARBS	81 g
	FIBER	3 g			FIBER	3 g
	SUGAR	14 g			SUGAR	19 g
	SODIUM	1,090 mg			SODIUM	2,520 mg
	PROTEIN	24 g			PROTEIN	53 g

Grilled Chicken Salad with Low-Fat Balsamic Vinaigrette	SERVING	1 order		Southwest Grilled Chicken Salad with Chipotle Caesar Dressing	SERVING	1 order
	CALORIES	285			CALORIES	710
	FAT	19.5 g			FAT	50 g
	CARBS	19 g	Save **425** calories		CARBS	29 g
	FIBER	4 g			FIBER	6 g
	SUGAR	11 g			SUGAR	7 g
	SODIUM	1,070 mg			SODIUM	1,950 mg
	PROTEIN	29 g			PROTEIN	37 g

TIP Reach for orange and yellow fruits and vegetables to reduce your risk of developing lung cancer by up to 25 percent. These foods get their color from **carotenoids**, cancer-fighting compounds. Increase the carotenoids in your diet by snacking on red, yellow and orange peppers, oranges, mangoes, carrots, tangerines, sweet potatoes and peaches.

EVEN BETTER

Chicken is a good source of vitamin B6: four ounces of chicken will supply about one-third of a person's daily needs for vitamin B6. In addition to its role in energy metabolism, vitamin B6 prevents the dangerous molecule, homocysteine, from accumulating. This molecule is so damaging to blood vessel walls that high levels of it are considered a significant risk factor for cardiovascular disease.

BONUS!

Researchers have found that eating chicken can help protect against Alzheimer's and age-related cognitive decline. Regular consumption of foods that are rich in the nutrient niacin, such as chicken, can provide protection against these conditions.

PICK IT ✓   KICK IT ✗

Bottomless Tostada Chips with Salsa	SERVING	1 order		Loaded Beef Nachos	SERVING	1 order
	CALORIES	480			CALORIES	1,150
	FAT	29 g			FAT	82 g
	CARBS	36 g	Save 2,570 mg sodium		CARBS	42 g
	FIBER	4 g			FIBER	8 g
	SUGAR	0 g			SUGAR	0 g
	SODIUM	2,050 mg			SODIUM	4,620 mg
	PROTEIN	5 g			PROTEIN	91 g

GG Grilled Chicken Sandwich with Veggies	SERVING	1 order		Southern Smokehouse Burger with Ancho Chile BBQ	SERVING	1 order
	CALORIES	610			CALORIES	2,080
	FAT	12 g			FAT	147 g
	CARBS	78 g	Save 1,470 calories		CARBS	141 g
	FIBER	8 g			FIBER	10 g
	SUGAR	0 g			SUGAR	0 g
	SODIUM	1,310 mg			SODIUM	6,060 mg
	PROTEIN	44 g			PROTEIN	91 g

YES YOU CAN

Drink alcohol and be healthy! **Moderate consumption of alcohol lowers the risk of developing heart disease and diabetes but slightly increases the risk of developing breast and colon cancer.** Opt for an occasional drink as a treat instead of indulging frequently.

BONUS!

Beef is packed with high-quality protein and is a great source of iron and zinc, minerals many Americans have trouble getting. Eating meat makes it much easier to get these much-needed minerals and eating lean meat is also a superb way to get vitamin B12, niacin and vitamin B6.

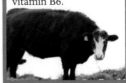

70

Percentage of adults who said they are more likely to visit a restaurant that offers locally produced food items.

– National Restaurant Association 2009 Restaurant Industry Forecast

PICK IT ✓   # KICK IT ✗

Veggie Cheese Omelet	SERVING	1 order	All-American Slam	SERVING	1 order
	CALORIES	500		CALORIES	820
	FAT	37 g		FAT	69 g
	CARBS	10 g		CARBS	5 g
	FIBER	2 g		FIBER	1 g
	SUGAR	4 g		SUGAR	1 g
	SODIUM	940 mg		SODIUM	1,520 mg
	PROTEIN	29 g		PROTEIN	42 g

Save 580 mg sodium

Country Fried Steak and Eggs	SERVING	1 order	Country Fried Steak with Gravy	SERVING	1 order
	CALORIES	660		CALORIES	1,000
	FAT	42 g		FAT	65 g
	CARBS	29 g		CARBS	54 g
	FIBER	3 g		FIBER	6 g
	SUGAR	0 g		SUGAR	1 g
	SODIUM	1,420 mg		SODIUM	2,580 mg
	PROTEIN	39 g		PROTEIN	51 g

Save 1,160 mg sodium

EXCUSE BUSTED

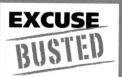

Want to hang out with your friends instead of exercising?

Get friends who exercise! A survey of nearly 1,000 college students found that men who have friends who exercise are more likely to exercise as well.

FATTER, NOT FITTER

Overestimating how much food your body needs is among the most common weight-maintenance mistakes, experts say. Be aware of portion sizes! Weigh and measure standard portions, at least at first, so you'll know what the amounts should look like. And never use restaurant portions as your guide – they super-size everything.

BONUS!

Eating veggies

can lower your risk of developing type 2 diabetes. Type 2 diabetes affects over 12 million people and causes more than 140,000 deaths in the United States each year. It also significantly increases your risk for heart disease, kidney disease, blindness and amputations.

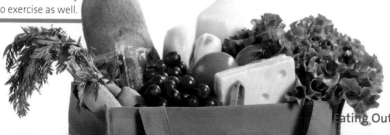

Eating Out At *DOMINO'S*

PICK IT ✓ KICK IT ✗

Hand Tossed 14" Large with Ham		
SERVING	1 slice
CALORIES	255
FAT	8.5 g
CARBS	34 g
FIBER	2 g
SUGAR	3 g
SODIUM	625 mg
PROTEIN	12 g

Save 465 mg sodium

Deep dish 14" Large Pepperoni Feast		
SERVING	1 slice
CALORIES	410
FAT	22 g
CARBS	42 g
FIBER	5 g
SUGAR	2 g
SODIUM	1,090 mg
PROTEIN	16 g

Thin Crust 14" Large Veggie Feast		
SERVING	1 slice
CALORIES	270
FAT	10.5 g
CARBS	36 g
FIBER	2 g
SUGAR	2 g
SODIUM	650 mg
PROTEIN	13 g

Choose thin crust and save an extra 54 calories!

Save 490 mg sodium

Deep Dish Large Meatzza Feast		
SERVING	1 slice
CALORIES	430
FAT	22 g
CARBS	42 g
FIBER	5 g
SUGAR	2 g
SODIUM	1,140 mg
PROTEIN	18 g

Eating Out At *JACK IN THE BOX*

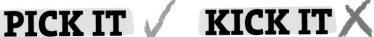

PICK IT ✓ KICK IT ✗

Hamburger Deluxe		
SERVING	1 order
CALORIES	340
FAT	18 g
CARBS	31 g
FIBER	2 g
SUGAR	6 g
SODIUM	550 mg
PROTEIN	14 g

Save 1,330 mg sodium

Bacon Ultimate Cheeseburger		
SERVING	1 order
CALORIES	980
FAT	67 g
CARBS	52 g
FIBER	2 g
SUGAR	11 g
SODIUM	1,880 mg
PROTEIN	43 g

Fajita Chicken Pita		
SERVING	1 order
CALORIES	320
FAT	11 g
CARBS	33 g
FIBER	4 g
SUGAR	3 g
SODIUM	1,110 mg
PROTEIN	24 g

Save 400 calories

Homestyle Ranch Chicken Club		
SERVING	1 order
CALORIES	720
FAT	33 g
CARBS	74 g
FIBER	3 g
SUGAR	9 g
SODIUM	1,860 mg
PROTEIN	33 g

Stock up on veggies for a healthy heart! Researchers are serving up further proof that eating fruits and vegetables is good for you. Vegetarians were found to have higher blood levels of salicylic acid, an anti-inflammatory present in fruits and vegetables. Researchers believe the high concentration of salicylic acid in these foods may help explain other studies that revealed low levels of heart disease among people who eat lots of these good-for-you foods.

YES YOU CAN

COOK AT HOME:

Cook a big batch of mixed vegetables (steam or roast) and add them to your meals all week long.

TOP CHOICE!
Eat garlic for better overall health! Two reviews of studies examining the effects of garlic suggest that not only is it good for the heart, it may also help ward off stomach and colon cancers. You don't need to eat garlic every day; five cloves of raw or cooked garlic per week is sufficient.

SAY WHAT? What you crave may indicate how you feel. Researchers found women crave food more often than men do, with cravings increasing during times of low mood or anxiety. Chocolate cravings may be a signal that you are tired. An urge for salty foods or dairy products may be your body's way of telling you it wants a real meal.

Eating Out At KFC

PICK IT ✓   KICK IT ✗

Toasted Wrap with Oven Roasted Strip and Large Corn on the Cob			Crispy Twister with Crispy Strips and Mashed Potatoes with Gravy		
SERVING	1 serving			**SERVING**	1 serving
CALORIES	378			**CALORIES**	710
FAT	14.5 g			**FAT**	34.5 g
CARBS	40 g			**CARBS**	69 g
FIBER	2.9 g			**FIBER**	4 g
SUGAR	4.4 g			**SUGAR**	5 g
SODIUM	742 mg			**SODIUM**	1,800 mg
PROTEIN	24.4 g			**PROTEIN**	30 g

Save 1,058 mg sodium

Honey BBQ Sandwich and Seasoned Rice			Rice and Gravy Famous Bowl		
SERVING	1 order			**SERVING**	1 order
CALORIES	450			**CALORIES**	790
FAT	4.5 g			**FAT**	28 g
CARBS	73 g			**CARBS**	106 g
FIBER	2 g			**FIBER**	5 g
SUGAR	20 g			**SUGAR**	4 g
SODIUM	1,370 mg			**SODIUM**	2,690 mg
PROTEIN	26 g			**PROTEIN**	29 g

Save 340 calories

A side order of coleslaw has less than half the sodium of seasoned rice — only 270 mg.

BONUS!

Corn is great

fuel for a healthy heart, partly because it contains folate. Folate helps lower levels of homocysteine, which can directly damage blood vessels, so elevated blood levels of this dangerous molecule are a risk factor for heart attack, stroke and peripheral vascular disease.

≫ FAST FACT

It is estimated that if we each consumed 100 percent of the daily value of folate, this alone would reduce the number of heart attacks suffered by Americans each year by 10 percent. Folate-rich diets are also associated with a reduced risk of developing colon cancer. A cup of corn supplies 19 percent of the daily value for folate.

Try This

Antioxidants such as vitamins E and C, selenium and lycopene play a significant role in preventing diseases such as cancer and heart disease. To benefit from antioxidants, eat a wide variety of fruits and vegetables — the more colorful the better!

PICK IT ✓ KICK IT ✗

Freshside Grille Smart Choice Shrimp Scampi				Popcorn Shrimp		
	SERVING	1 order			SERVING	1 order
	CALORIES	110			CALORIES	270
	FAT	5 g			FAT	16 g
	CARBS	1 g	*Save* **160** calories		CARBS	23 g
	FIBER	0 g			FIBER	1 g
	SUGAR	0 g			SUGAR	1 g
	SODIUM	610 mg			SODIUM	570 mg
	PROTEIN	18 g			PROTEIN	9 g
Grilled Pacific Salmon				Battered Fish		
	SERVING	1 order			SERVING	1 order
	CALORIES	150			CALORIES	520
	FAT	5 g			FAT	32 g
	CARBS	2 g	*Save* **370** calories		CARBS	34 g
	FIBER	0 g			FIBER	0 g
	SUGAR	1 g			SUGAR	0 g
	SODIUM	440 mg			SODIUM	1,580 mg
	PROTEIN	24 g			PROTEIN	24 g

BONUS!

Salmon is low in

calories and saturated fat, yet higher in omega-3 fatty acids than most other fish. The fat composition of salmon helps reduce risk of unwanted inflammation and help maintain immune and circulatory systems.

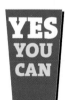

YES YOU CAN

Get in those antioxidants for a healthier you! Antioxidants are believed to provide a protective effect against conditions such as heart disease and cancer by interfering with the damage caused by free radicals. Antioxidants are also believed to help retard the aging process. Reach for those prunes, raisins, blueberries, blackberries, kale, strawberries and spinach to eat and live well.

Say What?

ENJOYING SALMON just twice a week may help raise omega-3 levels as effectively as (if not more than) daily fish oil supplementation, according to a study published in the *American Journal of Clinical Nutrition*.

 FAST FACT
More adult American women are obese (33 percent) than men (28 percent).

PICK IT ✓   KICK IT ✗

Quarter Pounder (No Cheese)				Big Mac		
	SERVING	1 order			SERVING	1 order
	CALORIES	410			CALORIES	540
	FAT	19 g	*Save 130 calories*		FAT	29 g
	CARBS	37 g			CARBS	45 g
	FIBER	2 g			FIBER	3 g
	SUGAR	8 g			SUGAR	9 g
	SODIUM	730 mg			SODIUM	1,040 mg
	PROTEIN	24 g			PROTEIN	25 g

Premium Caesar Salad with Grilled Chicken (No Dressing)				Premium Southwest Salad with Crispy Chicken and Southwest Dressing		
	SERVING	1 salad			SERVING	1 salad and 1 packet of dressing
	CALORIES	220	*Save 310 calories*		CALORIES	530
	FAT	6 g			FAT	26 g
	CARBS	12 g			CARBS	49 g
	FIBER	3 g			FIBER	6 g
	SUGAR	5 g			SUGAR	15 g
	SODIUM	890 g			SODIUM	1,260 mg
	PROTEIN	30 g			PROTEIN	27 g

FATTER, NOT FITTER

While a chicken breast has less than half the fat of a steak and the fat is less saturated, **eating chicken with the skin on doubles the amount of fat and saturated fat. For this reason, chicken is best skinned before eating.**

TIP Get enough protein for overall health, hormonal balance, muscle repair and immune system function. Eating protein can also help you lose weight: it triggers the secretion of a hormone called glucagon, which helps you break down fat. *Good sources of protein include 3 oz (1/2 can) of tuna = 22 g, 4 oz of chicken = 28 g, 1/2 cup of tofu = 20 g, 1/2 cup of cottage cheese = 15 g.*

YES YOU CAN! Get the following nutrients every day: low-glycemic-index carbohydrates (whole grains, fruits, vegetables and beans), vitamin C (broccoli, mangos and oranges) and vitamin D (from supplements, from the sun and from food such as salmon, sardines, shrimp, milk, cod and eggs).

Eating Out At OLIVE GARDEN

PICK IT ✓ KICK IT ✗

Linguini Alla Marinara			Spaghetti and Italian Sausage		
SERVING	1 order		SERVING	1 order	
CALORIES	551		CALORIES	1,270	
FAT	8 g		FAT	61 g	
CARBS	79 g	Save 2,320 mg sodium	CARBS	97 g	
FIBER	8 g		FIBER	15 g	
SUGAR	0 g		SUGAR	0 g	
SODIUM	770 mg		SODIUM	3,090 mg	
PROTEIN	14 g		PROTEIN	66.5 g	

Parmesan Crusted Tilapia			Seafood Alfredo		
SERVING	1 order		SERVING	1 order	
CALORIES	753		CALORIES	1,046	
FAT	25.2 g		FAT	55 g	
CARBS	87.3 g	Save 702 mg sodium	CARBS	98 g	
FIBER	13.5 g		FIBER	0 g	
SUGAR	8.2 g		SUGAR	0 g	
SODIUM	1,728 mg		SODIUM	2,430 mg	
PROTEIN	50 g		PROTEIN	44.3 g	

 FAST FACT

A healthy diet can prevent or even reverse four out of the six leading causes of death in the U.S.! Evidence indicates that diet is more important than genetics in the vast majority of cases of heart disease, stroke, cancer and type 2 diabetes.

Carbohydrates

BONUS!

such as whole wheat or whole grain pasta provide glucose, essential fuel for your brain and muscles. Pasta is also an excellent source of complex carbohydrates, which provide a slow release of energy, unlike simple sugars.

TOP CHOICE! *Tilapia*

Tilapia is a great nutritious option. A three-ounce serving (85 grams) of tilapia contains 80 calories, 16 grams of protein, and one-and-a-half grams of fat, with no saturated and trans fats. It is an excellent source of niacin, vitamin B12, potassium, selenium and phosphorus.

Say What?

DON'T CUT OUT CARBS. Experts say you should never cut any food group out of your diet — including carbohydrates. Equally important is to learn which carbohydrates give you the biggest bang for your nutritional buck. Go for foods rich in healthy complex carbs, such as fresh fruits, vegetables and whole grains.

PICK IT ✓   KICK IT ✗

Outback Special Steak (6 oz) with Steamed Green Beans and Baked Sweet Potato (All Without Butter or Seasoning)			Prime Rib (8 oz) with Caesar Salad and Garlic Mashed Potatoes		
	SERVING	1 serving		SERVING	1 serving
	CALORIES	555		CALORIES	1,549
	FAT	12.7 g		FAT	134 g
	CARBS	63.5 g		CARBS	59.6 g
	FIBER	11.2 g		FIBER	7.3 g
	SUGAR	9.6 g		SUGAR	1 g
	SODIUM	2,451 mg		SODIUM	3,709 mg
	PROTEIN	45.7 g		PROTEIN	47.9 g

Save 994 calories

Classic Cheesecake (No Sauce)			Nutter Butter Peanut Butter Pie		
	SERVING	1 serving		SERVING	1 serving
	CALORIES	737		CALORIES	1,760
	FAT	54 g		FAT	112.8 g
	CARBS	104.7 g		CARBS	177.8 g
	FIBER	1.3 g		FIBER	5 g
	SUGAR	50.4 g		SUGAR	68 g
	SODIUM	332.5 mg		SODIUM	1,347 mg
	PROTEIN	8.5 g		PROTEIN	24.9 g

Save 1,023 calories

Try This!

Take your time chewing all of your meals. When asked why you're a slowpoke, tell your family that enjoying your food takes time and prevents you from eating too much. In a Japanese study involving more than 3,000 men and women, people who reported eating quickly were three times more likely to be fat than people who ate more slowly. Why? Quick eaters shovel more into their mouths in an attempt to feel full. Researchers suspect fast eating could be triggered by mental stress, which then drives people to eat high-calorie foods, another reason they may be overweight.

BETTER CHOICE

Salsa isn't just fat free and nutrient rich – it's also versatile. You can use it as a dip, sauce or salad dressing – it even tastes great in a sandwich or wrap filled with lettuce, cucumbers and chicken. It's also a tasty topping for grilled meats, eggs or beans.

PICK IT ✓ KICK IT ✗

Naked Chicken Strips and Biscuit		
SERVING	1 order
CALORIES	460
FAT	23 g
CARBS	28 g
FIBER	1 g
SUGAR	2 g
SODIUM	1,210 mg
PROTEIN	34 g

Ditch the biscuit and save 490 mg of sodium!

Save 490 mg sodium

Mild Chicken Breast and Mashed Potatoes and Gravy		
SERVING	1 order
CALORIES	470
FAT	24 g
CARBS	26 g
FIBER	2 g
SUGAR	0 g
SODIUM	1,700 mg
PROTEIN	26 g

Po Boy Sandwich		
SERVING	1 order
CALORIES	330
FAT	17 g
CARBS	36 g
FIBER	0 g
SUGAR	10 g
SODIUM	560 mg
PROTEIN	8 g

Order yours with a side of green beans!

Save 300 calories

Deluxe Mild or Spicy with Mayo		
SERVING	1 order
CALORIES	630
FAT	31 g
CARBS	53 g
FIBER	3 g
SUGAR	5 g
SODIUM	1,480 mg
PROTEIN	35 g

ALL YOU!

Experiencing hot flashes? You may have low bone mineral density. According to a recent study published in the journal *Menopause*, women who suffer from hot flashes or night sweats have lower bone mineral density than women with no symptoms. If you have lower bone mineral density, you can develop weaker bones that can lead to fractures. You can increase your bone density by taking vitamin D and calcium supplements and fitting in weight-training exercises.

TIP Boost your magnesium intake to help lower your risk of developing diabetes by 10 to 34 percent. Studies have shown that eating foods rich in magnesium is a good way to help your body regulate insulin. Magnesium-rich foods include nuts, black beans, whole grains, dried fruits and leafy green vegetables.

YES YOU CAN

Stay hydrated. Drinking eight glasses of water a day not only fills you up, it also increases your energy, flushes out waste and provides fluoride for your teeth. Dehydration can lead to exhaustion and an energy slump in the latter half of your day. How can you commit to drinking eight glasses a day? Fill up a large bottle each morning and drink it by the day's end.

Eating Out At SUBWAY

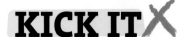

PICK IT ✓   KICK IT ✗

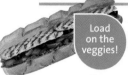

Load on the veggies!

6" Oven Roasted Chicken Sandwich

SERVING	1 order	
CALORIES	319	
FAT	4.5 g	**Save 787 mg** sodium
CARBS	48.4 g	
FIBER	5.5 g	
SUGAR	7 g	
SODIUM	743 mg	
PROTEIN	23 g	

6" Meatball Marinara Sandwich

SERVING	1 order
CALORIES	560
FAT	23 g
CARBS	70 g
FIBER	9 g
SUGAR	16 g
SODIUM	1,530 mg
PROTEIN	24 g

Chicken Tortilla Soup

SERVING	1 order	
CALORIES	110	
FAT	1.5 g	
CARBS	11 g	**Save 30** calories
FIBER	3 g	
SUGAR	4 g	
SODIUM	440 mg	
PROTEIN	6 g	

Chipotle Chicken Corn Chowder

SERVING	1 order
CALORIES	140
FAT	3 g
CARBS	22 g
FIBER	2 g
SUGAR	4 g
SODIUM	900 mg
PROTEIN	6 g

Eating Out At TACO BELL

PICK IT ✓   KICK IT ✗

Steak Gordita Supreme

SERVING	1 gordita	
CALORIES	300	
FAT	14 g	
CARBS	30 g	**Save 1,380 mg** sodium
FIBER	3 g	
SUGAR	6 g	
SODIUM	630 mg	
PROTEIN	14 g	

Volcano Burrito

SERVING	1 burrito
CALORIES	800
FAT	42 g
CARBS	41 g
FIBER	8 g
SUGAR	6 g
SODIUM	2,010 mg
PROTEIN	24 g

Triple Layer Nachos

Choose nachos with beans to save calories, fat and sodium!

SERVING	1 order	
CALORIES	340	
FAT	18 g	
CARBS	38 g	**Save 420** calories
FIBER	6 g	
SUGAR	2 g	
SODIUM	720 mg	
PROTEIN	7 g	

Nachos Bell Grande

SERVING	1 order
CALORIES	760
FAT	42 g
CARBS	77 g
FIBER	12 g
SUGAR	5 g
SODIUM	1,250 mg
PROTEIN	19 g

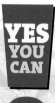

YES YOU CAN

Exercise your way to a healthier stomach! Researchers studied the effect of exercise in a survey of more than 11,000 people. Men who were moderately active – defined as walking or jogging up to 10 miles per week, or equivalent activity – had 46 percent less risk of developing stomach ulcers than their sedentary counterparts.

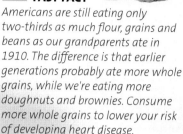

 FAST FACT

Americans are still eating only two-thirds as much flour, grains and beans as our grandparents ate in 1910. The difference is that earlier generations probably ate more whole grains, while we're eating more doughnuts and brownies. Consume more whole grains to lower your risk of developing heart disease.

BONUS!

Beef contains heme iron, a highly usable form of iron that is easily absorbed by your body. What's more, eating meat enhances the absorption of nonheme iron from plant foods. That's a good reason to use smaller portions of meat mixed with plant foods in your meals. What's more, the zinc in meat is absorbed better than the zinc in grains and legumes.

COOK AT HOME:

FLANK STEAK – pair it with a salad to boost your intake of veggies.

SAY WHAT? Pick up those weights to lose some weight! A new study found that strength training plays an important role in getting rid of extra weight. Aerobic exercise may burn calories, but the body's metabolism quickly returns to pre-exercise levels, usually within 30 minutes or so. According to researchers at Johns Hopkins University, resistance training leads to increased calorie burning for up to two hours after the workout is over.

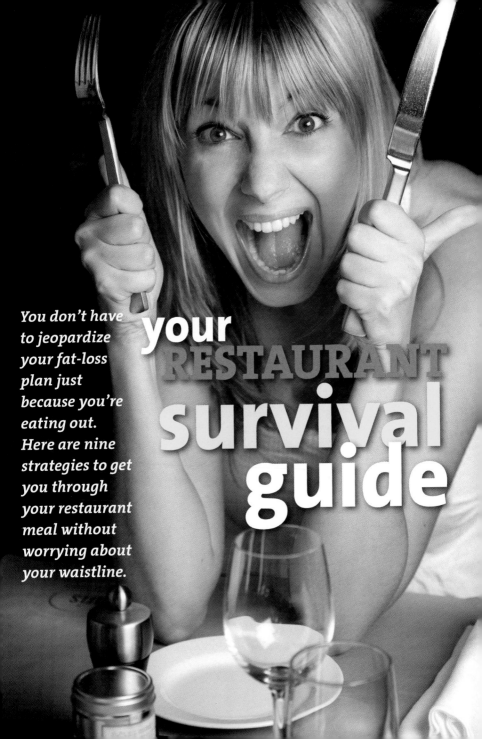

You don't have to jeopardize your fat-loss plan just because you're eating out. Here are nine strategies to get you through your restaurant meal without worrying about your waistline.

your
RESTAURANT
survival
guide

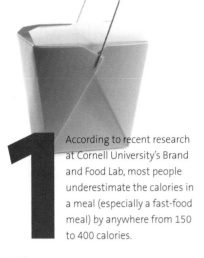

1 According to recent research at Cornell University's Brand and Food Lab, most people underestimate the calories in a meal (especially a fast-food meal) by anywhere from 150 to 400 calories.

TIP: *Stick to restaurants known for their healthy food options. When the meal arrives, eat only half. Share it with your date or take the other half home with you for tomorrow's lunch.*

2 The proper "visual cue" for a portion of salad dressing is the size of a standard shot glass. "The typical shot glass contains one and a half ounces, which would be an appropriate amount of salad dressing to use," says Lisa Young, PhD, RD, author of *The Portion Teller Plan* (Morgan Road Books, 2006). "One ounce is equivalent to approximately two tablespoons, but restaurants typically give at least double this amount." **Translation: twice the fat.**

TIP: *To cut down on fat intake, order low-fat salad dressing on the side, and then dip your fork between bites to get the flavor without tons of extra fat.*

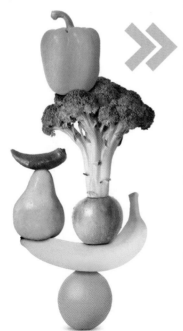

3 If you're following the USDA's recommendation to eat seven to ten servings of vegetables and fruit daily, you no doubt know that drinking juice counts toward your total. However, most people don't know how many calories juice contains, according to Esther Blum, RD, holistic nutritionist and author of *Eat, Drink, and Be Gorgeous* (Chronicle Books, 2007). A cup of orange juice contains the same number of calories as an equivalent amount of Coca-Cola (although it's packed with significantly more nutrients per serving). And four ounces is the correct serving size. Yes, only half a cup!

TIP: *To cut calories while keeping taste and nutrition, mix your OJ with an equal amount of mineral water, plain water or seltzer, and then give half to your dining companion. Do the same with most fruit juices.*

4

Over the last few years of supersizing portions, a typical bagel has doubled in size and more than doubled in calories. And that adds up quickly around your midsection and derriere.

TIP: *Eat only half the bagel and save the rest for later. You should, become conscious of portion sizes as matter of lifestyle choice, whether you eat at home or out on the town. And avoid most muffins — even low-fat versions will likely contain too much of the bad stuff. To offset the reduced fat content, the sugar levels will likely have been bumped up considerably.*

5

Artificial sweeteners may save you calories when you consume the product, but according to animal studies, there may be a downside later on. Researchers suggest that the body learns to associate sweetness with calories, but the use of artificial sweeteners makes the body less able to perform this juggling act.

TIP: *While the artificial sweetener industry claims that studies on animals have no relevance to humans, it's best to play it safe. When you're in a restaurant, ask for honey to sweeten your tea or coffee, and then use only a half-teaspoon's worth.*

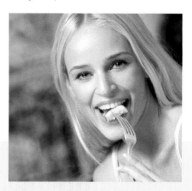

6

Eating meals quickly and without thought can lead to more fat gain, because we continue eating beyond what the body can process into energy.

TIP: *Because it can take your digestive tract up to 20 minutes to realize that you've supplied enough food to meet your body's needs, chew your food thoroughly and slow down. (See more on mindful eating in chapter three, page 118.)*

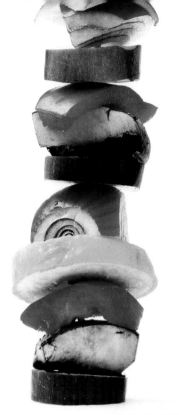

8 Anything "creamed," "scalloped," "au gratin," "sauteed" or "breaded" will likely be loaded with tons of fat, while foods that are "smoked" or "barbecued" (also those that are coated with teriyaki sauce) are packed with sodium, which will not only raise your blood pressure, but will also make you retain a significant amount of water.

TIP: *Always order "roasted," "grilled" or "broiled" foods, adding that you'd like them prepared plain, without any added butter, sauces or fats.*

9 Think of buffets as fat-laden traps. When foods are prepared in bulk, they are slathered in oil. And the way the buffet is displayed can tempt you into making all the wrong choices.

TIP: *If you must dine buffet-style, here's how to do it: Walk around the buffet, looking for clean eats such as lean protein sources (check the carving station), steamed vegetables, lettuce, cucumbers, tomatoes and other freshly cut water-rich vegetables, and fresh fruit). Next, grab a small plate, not a standard dinner-size plate, and pick appropriately sized portions of the clean foods you've spotted earlier. Skip breads and pastas, fried fare and foods floating in sauces. Avoid the salad dressings (use lemon). Drink plain or mineral water, or unsweetened tea. Eat slowly (see number six), and leave feeling satisfied but not stuffed.*

7 Don't "save your calories" by skipping meals or eating too lightly when you know you'll be going out later. Not only will you slow down your metabolism with this approach, you'll arrive at the dinner table famished, making you more likely to overeat.

TIP: *Start with a nutritious breakfast — it's the most important meal of the day. Continue eating clean all day long to maintain your fat-burning process.*

EATING OUT?
Get what you want

❶ GO WHERE THE SERVING STAFF KNOWS you. Get to know them and they're more likely to direct you to what's freshest and best for your waistline.

❷ ASK WHAT THE CHEF CAN GRILL OR poach; order a grilled or poached piece of fish or chicken with fresh herbs. Ask for substitutions – if the dish comes only with a cream sauce, for example, ask them if they'd mind using tomato sauce – chances are, they won't mind.

❸ CHOOSE A DISH THAT'S NATURALLY low in fat to start – don't take a fried item and try to make it healthier. Cultivate a taste for grilled chicken or shrimp and you'll soon want nothing but grilled or steamed, not fried.

❹ BEWARE OF THE CALORIES IN beverages, which can add up quickly. (I always order water with a slice of lemon.)

❺ PASS ON THE CHIPS OR BREAD – if you want to add a side, ask for a green salad with dressing on the side. Feel like a potato? Ask for plain baked one, without butter or sour cream. (At home I always add a dollop of plain nonfat yogurt and some restaurants carry this item. It doesn't hurt to ask!)

❻ BEWARE OF INDIVIDUAL PIZZAS, WHICH are often enough for four people. If you have a craving for pizza, split it and a salad with your date – you'll save money too!

❼ ORDER DRESSING ON THE SIDE INSTEAD of asking them for a small amount of dressing – a small amount to the kitchen staff might still be a lot for your waistline.

❽ IF YOU'VE BEEN CRAVING CHICKEN Parmesan and won't be satisfied by a grilled chicken salad, order the Chicken Parmesan and eat half. Ask for the rest to be boxed up to take home for tomorrow's meal. Add a salad and you've got tomorrow's dinner!

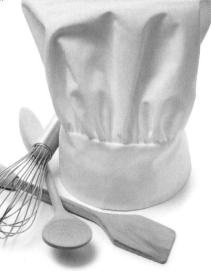

Menu
Keep In Mind

ASIAN RESTAURANTS

Order stir-fried chicken or fish and vegetables.

Ask for steamed rice instead of fried rice.

ITALIAN RESTAURANTS

Choose red sauces over white, creamy ones.

Order fish or pasta primavera instead of entrees with red meat.

Pass on the bread and grated Parmesan cheese.

MEXICAN RESTAURANTS

Choose salsa or picante sauce over sour cream or cheese.

Choose corn tortillas over flour ones.

Avoid refried beans.

•Go for a taco salad with grilled chicken and pass on the cheese and heavy sauces. If you crave guacamole, ask for it on the side and go easy.

Taken from American Heart Association *"What About Eating Out?"*

YOUR BEST & WORST
MENU PICKS!

When it comes to eating out, portion control is key – choose smarter foods (and less of them) and you'll bust fat without even knowing it!

PICK IT ✓   KICK IT ✗

CHINESE *Lots of dishes are deep fried and sauces are loaded with sugar.*

Steamed Dumplings	Low in fat.	*Crispy Noodles*	Lots of fat and may have trans fat.
Wonton Soup	Low in calories and filling.	*Spare Ribs*	Sugary sauce and fatty meat.
Tofu Dishes	Healthy protein.	*Egg Rolls*	High in calories and sodium.
Bamboo-Steamed Entrees	High in fiber and protein.	*Fried Rice*	High in fat and sodium.
Stir-Fry	Antioxidant-packed veggies. ASK FOR LESS OIL!	*Egg Foo Yung*	High in cholesterol and may have trans fat.

ITALIAN *Watch for large portions, fatty cream sauces and cheese overload.*

Love This!

Minestrone	Loaded with fiber and protein.	*Lasagna*	High in calories and oversized portions.
Whole Wheat Pasta with Marinara Sauce	Low in cholesterol with lots of vitamins.	*Alfredo*	High in saturated fat and sodium.
Thin-Crust Pizza	Less carbs and less calories.	*Thick Crust Pizza*	Extra carbs and calories.
Antipasto Grilled Veggies	Antioxidants and good fats.	*Meat Sauce*	High in saturated fat.

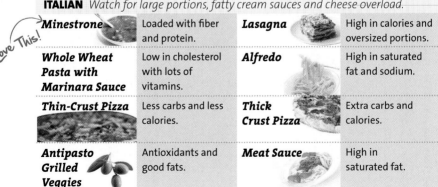

PICK IT ✓ KICK IT ✗

JAPANESE *Use caution with tempura and fried noodles.*

Sushi and Nigiri	Lean fish and steamed rice are clean eats.	**Tempura**	Fat, fat and more fat!
Sashimi	Omega-3 fats and protein.	**Sake and Plum Wine**	Lots of calories come from alcohol and sugar.
Teppan Yaki	Steak, seafood and vegetables — a well-balanced dish.	**Sukiyaki**	Made with lard and sugar, high in cholesterol.
Teriyaki Chicken	Lean protein. ASK FOR SAUCE ON THE SIDE.	**Gyoza**	Fried and stuffed with pork, tons of saturated fat.

MEXICAN *Watch the fatty sour cream, deep-fried corn chips and processed cheese.*

Gazpacho	High in iron and vitamin C.	**Margaritas**	High in calories from sugar and alcohol.
Chicken Fajitas	Lean protein and antioxidant-rich veggies. PASS ON THE SOUR CREAM.	**Nachos**	High in saturated fat and sodium.
Burrito	Can be low in cholesterol.	**Refried Beans**	High in protein but way too much sodium.
Guacamole	Healthy fats – just limit yourself to one tablespoon.	**Quesadillas**	Can be high in saturated fat.

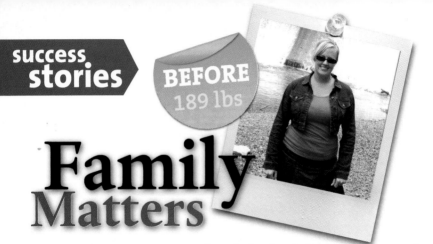

BEFORE
189 lbs

Family
Matters

When Allison Earnst realized she had three little people watching her every move, she decided to get into shape – and lost almost 60 lbs – for her family. BY KATHLEEN ENGEL

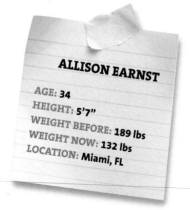

ALLISON EARNST

AGE: **34**

HEIGHT: **5'7"**

WEIGHT BEFORE: **189 lbs**

WEIGHT NOW: **132 lbs**

LOCATION: **Miami, FL**

"My body keeps responding the more I keep changing things."

A sk Allison Earnst her top tip for starting a fit lifestyle and she doesn't hesitate. "Find out what motivates you and you'll stick with it," she says.

For Allison, it was the realization that her three young children looked up to her. "If I eat a greasy cheeseburger and fries, they see that," she says. Six months after giving birth to her third child, Allison decided her days of fast food drive-thrus were over.

SMALL CHANGES

Placing a picture of *Oxygen* cover girl Jamie Eason on her fridge helped Allison commit to those first small changes. She started following *The Eat-Clean Diet* by Tosca Reno, stopped skipping breakfast and joined a gym. "I didn't go from one extreme to another," she says. Allison trained with a fitness model friend, working her entire body with three sets of weight training exercises. She also signed up for a body transformation challenge, knowing that short-term goals sustained her progress. Soon enough, she was eating six meals a day, carrying

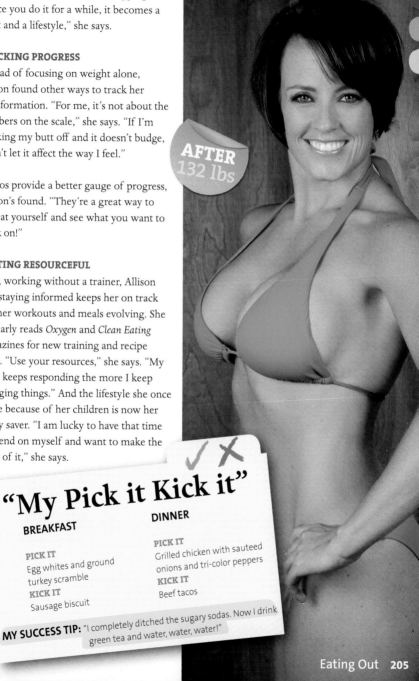

AFTER
132 lbs

around a protein shaker and dropping fat. "Once you do it for a while, it becomes a habit and a lifestyle," she says.

TRACKING PROGRESS

Instead of focusing on weight alone, Allison found other ways to track her transformation. "For me, it's not about the numbers on the scale," she says. "If I'm working my butt off and it doesn't budge, I don't let it affect the way I feel."

Photos provide a better gauge of progress, Allison's found. "They're a great way to look at yourself and see what you want to work on!"

GETTING RESOURCEFUL

Now, working without a trainer, Allison says staying informed keeps her on track and her workouts and meals evolving. She regularly reads *Oxygen* and *Clean Eating* magazines for new training and recipe ideas. "Use your resources," she says. "My body keeps responding the more I keep changing things." And the lifestyle she once chose because of her children is now her sanity saver. "I am lucky to have that time to spend on myself and want to make the most of it," she says.

"My Pick it Kick it"

BREAKFAST

PICK IT
Egg whites and ground turkey scramble
KICK IT
Sausage biscuit

DINNER

PICK IT
Grilled chicken with sauteed onions and tri-color peppers
KICK IT
Beef tacos

MY SUCCESS TIP: "I completely ditched the sugary sodas. Now I drink green tea and water, water, water!"

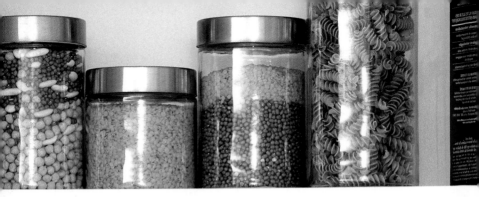

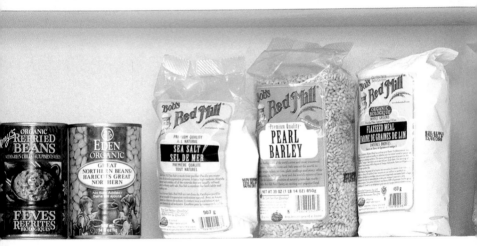

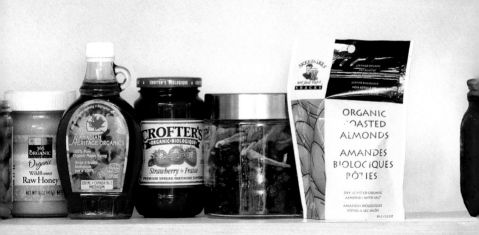

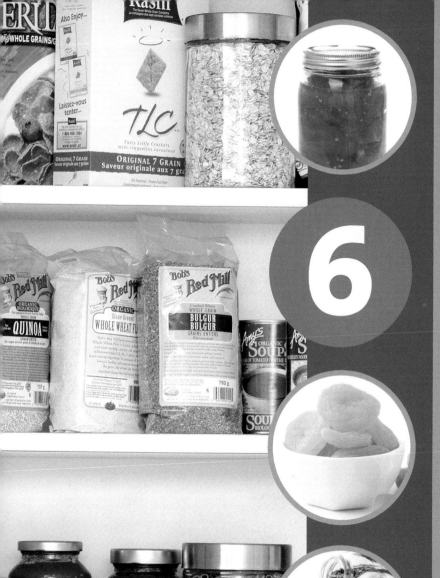

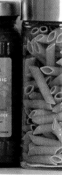

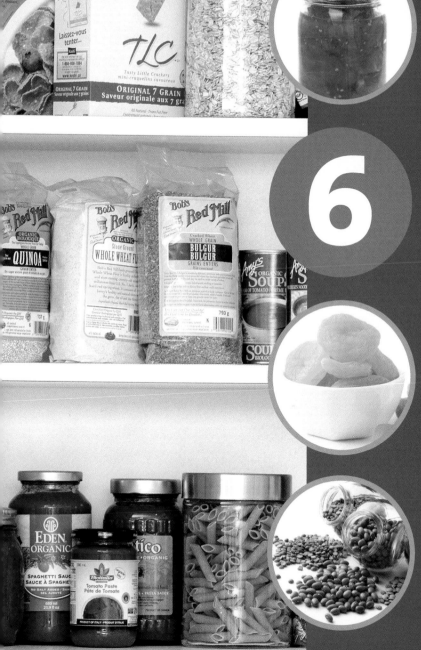

6

In Your Cupboard

"SHAPE up your KITCHEN"

STOCK YOUR SHELVES WITH FRESH, LOW-CAL FOOD – YOU'LL HAVE EASY WAYS TO DROP FAT WITHOUT EVEN THINKING ABOUT IT!

Losing fat isn't rocket science – eat fewer calories and you will drop pounds. But when you deprive yourself of some of your favorite foods, you may feel ticked off and eat even more … definitely not the way to success. A better and more sustainable method is to keep it simple. Swap a few high-fat, salty or sugary treats with healthier options and stock your pantry with them so they're the first things you reach for. Keep fruits and veggies at your fingertips on kitchen counters or on the kitchen table rather than decorating your house with dishes full of sweets. Goodbye, temptation!

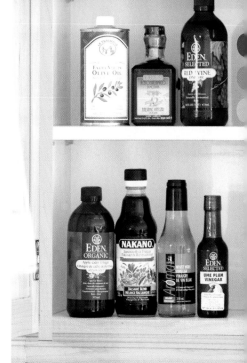

Make over your kitchen in tiny ways and cut out the little extras and you'll see results even during stressful times. I do my best to live a healthy life, but sometimes find myself straying off the *Oxygen* lifestyle path temporarily when I try to pack too much into my days. I've learned two key things: swapping out high-fat and sugary snacks really does work to keep my fat and stress levels down and the closer at hand fruits and veggies are, the more likely it is that I'll choose them when under stress.

One of the best ways you can lose fat is to dump all the temptations from your cupboards – a few simple swaps is all it takes! For example, I find myself habitually reaching for pita and hummus instead of chips and salsa – it's just as convenient. I only have balsamic vinegar and olive oil on hand for salad dressings. I put both bottles on the table and soon the kids were making their own creations by adding a dollop of Dijon mustard. Presto! Salad dressing that's fresh and nutritious! The key to it all? Reduce temptation. Shop wisely and stock your shelves with healthy food that's easy to reach for and simple to prepare.

"Make over your kitchen in tiny ways by cutting out the little extras and you'll see results even during stressful times"

PORTIONS MADE EASY

Cut this out and put it in your purse to use when you're not at home and near your measuring cups and spoons.

1 fist = 1 cup

1 palm = 3 ounces

1 thumb tip = 1 teaspoon

3 thumb tips = 1 tablespoon

1 thumb = 1 ounce of cheese

1 or 2 handfuls = 1 ounce of snack food

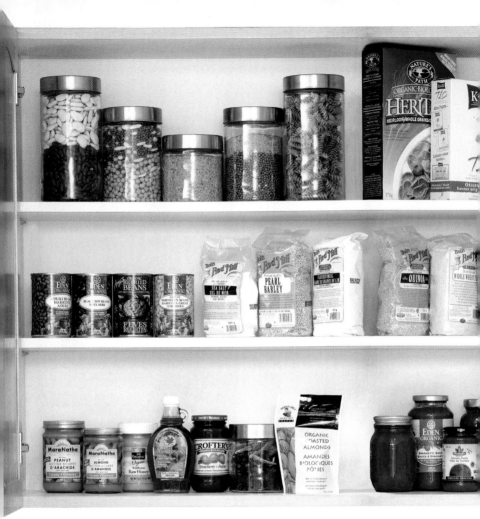

BUST FAT
With Your Groceries

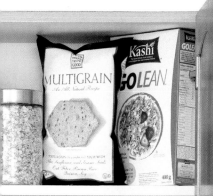

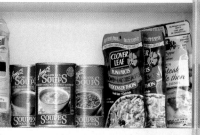

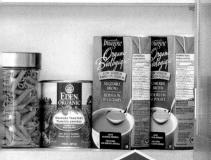

GO LOCAL. Not only will you save money, but some of the best-tasting produce is available at local markets because it is picked at peak flavor. It's also an eco-friendly way to shop!

PREP. When you get home from the store, spend 15 minutes washing and chopping all at once. Store your fruits and veggies in the fridge so they're easy to grab 'n' go.

EAT A SINGLE SERVING. Read the label to see the serving size, remove just that much and then put the package away. No eating directly out of the container — you will eat more than if you just take out small, portioned amounts.

SPICE IT UP. Avoid processed items such as seasoned rice packets. They are high in sodium and sometimes fat. You can easily buy plain brown rice and add your own seasoning.

PLAN FOR SNACK TIME. Be ready for a quick meal by stocking your pantry, car and office with a few staples: microwaveable soup and hot cereal, dried fruit, nuts and granola bars.

RAID THE REFRIGERATOR. Stock up on a variety of fresh vegetables for anytime noshing. Munching on a handful of baby carrots will meet your vitamin A needs for the entire day.

WHAT'S ALWAYS IN MY KITCHEN?

- steel cut oats
- low-fat plain yogurt
- unsweetened applesauce
- berries
- lemons
- tomatoes
- sea salt
- hummus
- popcorn
- artichoke hearts

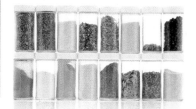

HOW TO START

Think of your pantry like your wardrobe. I am an avid pack rat – clothes I haven't worn for years are stuffed in the back of my closet. And guess what? They just take up space. So if you haven't used something in your cupboard in the past few weeks, toss it! Organizing your cupboards will make finding fresh, healthy items a breeze. Here's a checklist to get you started:

▶ First, clear off and wipe down the shelves. Just as you do when you're weeding out your closet, figure out what you never use and get rid of it.

▶ Place items you use all the time in the most accessible spots; items you use infrequently can go on the higher shelves or in the back.

▶ Store dry goods (beans, cereal, pasta, flour and rice) in containers with tight lids to keep out pests.

▶ Whole grains and milled whole grain products will last longer in the refrigerator or freezer (their natural oils tend to go rancid more rapidly at room temperature).

▶ Oils, especially olive oil and nut oils, should be kept on a dark shelf and away from heat to preserve their freshness and quality.

▶ Check condiments, seasonings, syrups and bottled cooking ingredients carefully – refrigeration may be necessary.

BEFORE RESTOCKING

Here's what you need to ask yourself before restocking your pantry:

1. Does the ingredients label and nutrition facts panel pass muster with my clean-eating plan? **Hint: Lots of ingredients with scientific names you can barely pronounce usually means a product is inappropriate.**

2. Do I have room for this item?

3. Have I used this at least once in the last six months? If not, keep it only if you have room.

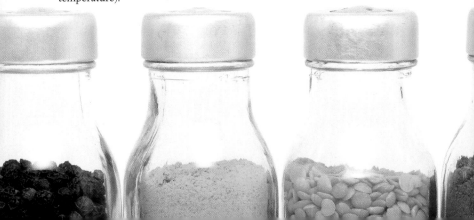

YOUR 3 PANTRY MUST-HAVES

Things you may not be eating but should (and they can easily be kept in your pantry).

FRESH OR CANNED PUMPKIN Pie is great, but pumpkin can be so much more! Pumpkin is rich in carotenoids — health-enhancing compounds that help maintain eye, lung and heart function.

Suggested Uses: Homemade pumpkin bread or pancakes are wonderful and nutritious, but also try a quick pumpkin "pudding" (pumpkin purée with low-fat plain yogurt and a dash of pumpkin pie spice, which includes cinnamon, ginger, nutmeg and allspice) or a savory pumpkin soup.

> BARLEY
> takes a while to cook (like most whole grains), so make a big batch, divide it and freeze it for later. Cooked barley will last for one week in the fridge or three months in the freezer.

PEARL BARLEY This grain boasts both soluble and insoluble fiber, so it keeps you feeling full, aids digestion, helps lower cholesterol and controls blood sugar response — all that, plus it has a healthy nutrition profile (low in fat, full of vitamins and minerals).

Suggested Uses: Serve it as a side dish (cook in low-sodium broth), in soups and stews, or as an alternative to rice or pasta in stir-fries and casseroles.

POUCH OR CANNED SALMON This is an at-the-ready alternative to your usual tuna and is an excellent source of omega-3 fatty acids, lean protein and even calcium if you leave in the bones (they're soft; just mash them with a fork). Opt for wild-caught salmon, if possible.

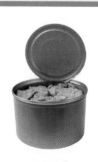

Suggested Uses: Try as a salad topper, casserole ingredient, or sandwich and wrap filler.

PICK IT

Nutritional Value

SERVING	2 Tbsp
CALORIES	20
FAT	0 g
CARBS	4 g
FIBER	0 g
SUGAR	4 g
SODIUM	10 mg
PROTEIN	0 g

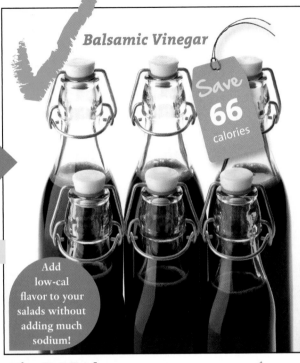

Balsamic Vinegar

Save **66** calories

Add low-cal flavor to your salads without adding much sodium!

BONUS!

Balsamic vinegar boosts activity of a digestive enzyme, pepsin, which in turn boosts metabolism. This means it's a great addition to your fat-loss cupboard! It has also been linked with reducing cholesterol and may help suppress your appetite.

Give It A Try!

Red wine vinegar (2 Tbsp)
6 calories, 0 fat, 2 mg sodium

Low-fat Italian dressing (2 Tbsp)
20 calories, 0.8 g fat, 600 mg sodium

Fat-free raspberry vinaigrette (2 Tbsp)
30 calories, 0 fat, 290 mg sodium

MAKE IT TONIGHT!

1 cup baby spinach
¼ cup celery, sliced
2 Tbsp carrot, shredded
1 Tbsp green onion, sliced
1 Tbsp homemade balsamic vinaigrette dressing (page right)

Makes 1 serving

YES YOU CAN

A versatile condiment, balsamic vinegar can be used in all kinds of dishes, including salads. But feel free to experiment – try it on proteins such as fish or eggs, or even sprinkled on fresh fruit such as strawberries, raspberries, blueberries or pears.

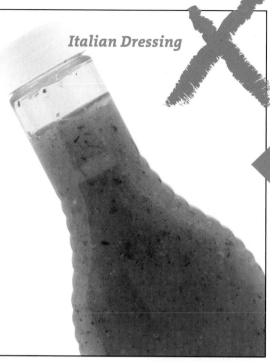
Italian Dressing

KICK IT

Nutritional Value

SERVING	2 Tbsp
CALORIES	86
FAT	8.3 g
CARBS	3.1 g
FIBER	0 g
SUGAR	2.4 g
SODIUM	486 mg
PROTEIN	2.1 g

❯ QUICK & EASY

Make your own easy vinaigrette by mixing ¼ cup olive oil, 2 Tbsp balsamic vinegar and 1 tsp Dijon mustard.

Ditch These Too!

Caesar dressing (2 Tbsp)
100 calories, 9 g fat, 240 mg sodium

Blue cheese dressing (2 Tbsp)
151 calories, 15.7 g fat, 328 mg sodium

Poppy seed dressing (2 Tbsp)
130 calories, 10 g fat, 250 mg sodium

Say What?

DID YOU know you can train your taste buds? Slowly reduce the sodium in your diet and over time you'll start preferring foods that taste less salty!

21

Percentage daily value of sodium in just two tablespoons of regular Italian dressing

Say What?

TRADITIONALLY, BALSAMIC VINEGAR is known for its healing properties. This vinegar has been so revered over the years that in many Italian families, new barrels of the best vinegars were started when a child was born and then given away at his or her future wedding.

PICK IT

Nutritional Value

SERVING	½ cup
CALORIES	40
FAT	0.2 g
CARBS	9 g
FIBER	1.8 g
SUGAR	5.2 g
SODIUM	642 mg
PROTEIN	1.6 g

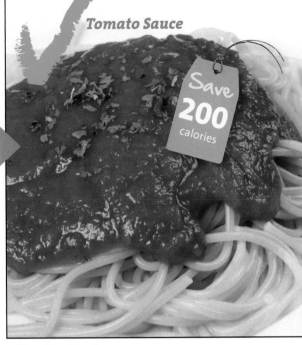

Tomato Sauce

Save **200** calories

MAKE IT BETTER

Choose low-sodium tomato sauce or make your own at home without adding any salt. Use herbs such as basil to add flavor the healthy way.

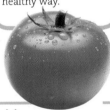

Give It a Try!

Low-fat mushroom and garlic pasta sauce (½ cup)
70 calories, 2 g fat, 260 mg sodium

Classico tomato and basil sauce (½ cup)
60 calories, 1 g fat, 310 mg sodium

Classico spicy red pepper sauce (½ cup)
60 calories, 1.5 g fat, 300 mg sodium

➤➤ FAST FACT

Tomatoes are a good source of potassium (lowers high blood pressure), niacin (lowers high cholesterol levels), Vitamin B6 and folate – it's a fruit that will keep your heart happy.

YES YOU CAN

Grow your own! Much like our First Lady Michelle Obama, you can discover the fresh taste and convenience of home-grown fruits and vegetables such as tomatoes by planting your own. Gardening can be a great way to save money – start small with some easy leafy greens and vegetables.

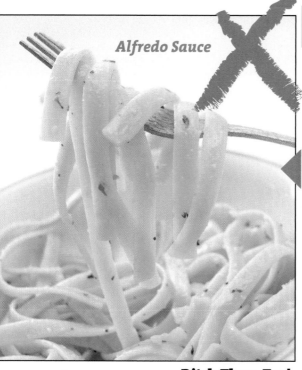

Alfredo Sauce

KICK IT

Nutritional Value	
SERVING	½ cup
CALORIES	240
FAT	22 g
CARBS	6 g
FIBER	0 g
SUGAR	2 g
SODIUM	760 mg
PROTEIN	4 g

> QUICK & EASY

Purée tomatoes, cucumbers, bell peppers and scallions in a blender and season with spices to make gazpacho, a refreshing cold soup, for a hot summer's dinner.

Ditch These Too!

Ragu spaghetti sauce (½ cup)
72 calories, 2.5 g fat, 480 mg sodium

Garden vegetable primavera (½ cup)
60 calories, 1 g fat, 610 mg sodium

Prego marinara pasta sauce (½ cup)
100 calories, 5 g fat, 550 mg sodium

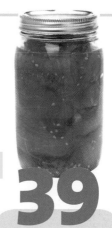

BONUS!

The antioxidant quality of lycopene, found in tomatoes, has been linked with everything from protecting cells to preventing heart disease and a host of cancers – prostate, breast, lung and pancreatic. Tomatoes are also packed with vitamins A and C and – most important for your fat-loss efforts – fiber, which has been shown to reduce cholesterol levels and keep blood sugar levels on an even keel.

39

Percentage daily value of Vitamin C in just one ripe tomato.

PICK IT

Salsa

love This!

Nutritional Value	
SERVING	2 Tbsp
CALORIES	23
FAT	0 g
CARBS	4.6 g
FIBER	0.6 g
SUGAR	3.4 g
SODIUM	538 mg
PROTEIN	1.1 g

Save **18** calories

Try salsa on your eggs, with your chicken dishes or in homemade burritos.

Give It A Try!

✓ **Fat-free sour cream (2 Tbsp)**
29 calories, 0.4 g fat, 23 mg sodium

✓ **Fat-free cream cheese (2 Tbsp)**
14 calories, 0.2 g fat, 79 mg sodium

✓ **Tzatziki (2 Tbsp)**
30 calories, 2.5 g fat, 25 mg sodium

QUICK & EASY

1 pound tomatoes, chopped

2 Tbsp chili peppers

6 green onions, chopped

1 cup cilantro, chopped

1 clove garlic

Sea salt to taste

Place in a blender or food processor until coarsely chopped. Serve with fish, meat, or as a sauce or dip. Keep refrigerated.

 FAST FACT *Salsa is a Spanish word for sauce. The main ingredients are tomatoes, garlic, onion and chilies. It is the number one condiment in the United States, replacing ketchup several years ago. (Remember that Seinfeld episode?)*

BONUS!

Salsa is loaded with vitamins A, B and C, as well as being a good source of iron, magnesium and potassium – important to keep blood pressure at a normal level.

Eat dips and sauces as part of your healthy lifestyle! Just remember to balance them with lots of fruits and vegetables, and eat them in moderation. Make better choices (such as salsa) and you'll see the benefits in a smaller waistline.

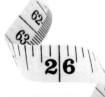

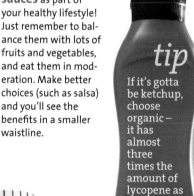

tip

If it's gotta be ketchup, choose organic – it has almost three times the amount of lycopene as non-organic versions.

SAY WHAT? In addition to the heart-healthy lycopene, salsa (made from tomatoes) also contains capsaicin, an anti-inflammatory linked to the prevention of ulcers and some cancers. But more important to your weight-loss efforts, capsaicin has a slight thermogenic quality, which may boost your metabolism.

KICK IT

Ketchup

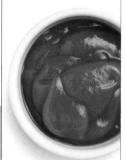

Nutritional Value

SERVING	2 Tbsp
CALORIES	41
FAT	0 g
CARBS	16.2 g
FIBER	0 g
SUGAR	8.1 g
SODIUM	608 mg
PROTEIN	0 g

Ditch These Too!

Honey, strained or extracted (2 Tbsp)
128 calories, 0 fat, 2 mg sodium

Barbecue sauce (2 Tbsp)
39 calories, 0.1 g fat, 424 mg sodium

Ranch dressing (2 Tbsp)
148 calories, 15.6 g fat, 287 mg sodium

PICK IT

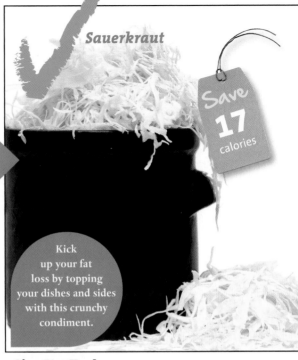

Sauerkraut

Save **17** calories

Nutritional Value

SERVING	2 Tbsp
CALORIES	22
FAT	0.1 g
CARBS	4.9 g
FIBER	2.8 g
SUGAR	2 g
SODIUM	760 mg
PROTEIN	1 g

Kick up your fat loss by topping your dishes and sides with this crunchy condiment.

Say What?

SAUERKRAUT, or fermented cabbage, was allegedly eaten by Dutch sailors on long sea trips to prevent scurvy.

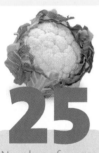

25

Number of grams of fiber you need every day. Many vegetables contain fiber, including cabbage, cauliflower and dark green leafy vegetables.

Give It a Try!

Classico sauce – fire-roasted tomato and garlic (2 Tbsp)
6 calories, 0 fat, 40 mg sodium ✓

Hummus (2 Tbsp)
54 calories, 2.6 g fat, 72 mg sodium ✓

Fat-free ranch dressing (2 Tbsp)
48 calories, 0.3 g fat, 354 mg sodium ✓

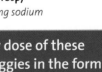

YES YOU CAN Add a daily dose of these wonder-veggies in the form of swiss chard, cabbage, broccoli, cauliflower, radishes, Brussel sprouts, arugula, spinach, turnip, watercress or rapini.

Sweet Pickle Relish

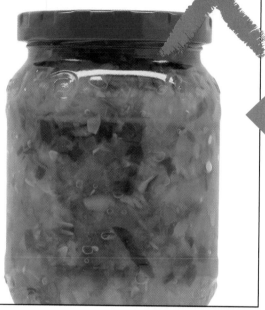

KICK IT

Nutritional Value	
SERVING	2 Tbsp
CALORIES	39
FAT	0.1 g
CARBS	10.2 g
FIBER	0.3 g
SUGAR	4.8 g
SODIUM	243 mg
PROTEIN	0.1 g

BONUS!

Cabbage
is also a goods source of Vitamin C, an antioxidant.

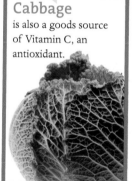

Ditch These Too!

Coleslaw (2 Tbsp)
24.5 calories, 1 g fat, 45 mg sodium

Honey mustard (2 Tbsp)
30 calories, 2 g fat, 75 mg sodium

Mayonnaise (2 Tbsp)
115 calories, 9.8 g fat, 209 mg sodium

Say What?

CABBAGE, the main ingredient in sauerkraut, is in the *Cruciferae* family of vegetables along with kale, broccoli, collards and Brussels sprouts. It's been linked in particular with better health for women. In fact, a study published in the journal *Cancer Research* cited the much lower risk of breast cancer in women who eat more vegetables from this family.

30
Number of pounds of cabbage and sauerkraut the average Polish woman eats every year, compared to just 10 pounds the average American woman eats every year.

PICK IT

Nutritional Value	
SERVING	2 Tbsp
CALORIES	14
FAT	0.2 g
CARBS	3.4 g
FIBER	1 g
SUGAR	2.4 g
SODIUM	94 mg
PROTEIN	0.4 g

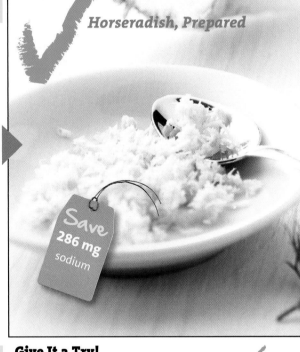

Horseradish, Prepared

Save 286 mg sodium

FATTER, NOT FITTER

Mayonnaise-type dressings are not only high in fat, they're also very high in sodium. Try horseradish instead if you're looking for a sharp hit of flavor.

BONUS!

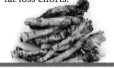

You get high taste impact with horseradish without the fat, a boost to your fat-loss efforts!

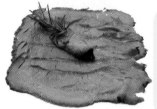

Give It a Try!

Chopped onions (2 Tbsp)
4 calories, 0 fat, 0 sodium ✓

Black pepper (1 tsp)
11 calories, 0.1 g fat, 2 mg sodium ✓

Miracle Whip nonfat dressing (2 Tbsp)
26 calories, 0.8 g fat, 252 mg sodium

Say What?

HORSERADISH (which uses a white root compared to a green root for wasabi) contains antioxidants important to women's health – vitamins E and C. Make great strides in your health simply by adding a few tablespoons of horseradish to your weekly diet. (It is an absolute must with roast beef!)

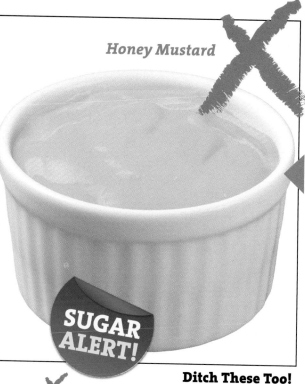

Honey Mustard

SUGAR ALERT!

KICK IT

Nutritional Value	
SERVING	2 Tbsp
CALORIES	60
FAT	0 g
CARBS	6 g
FIBER	0 g
SUGAR	3 g
SODIUM	180 mg
PROTEIN	0 g

Say What?

EVERY MAY, according to the Horseradish Information Council, there is an International Horseradish Festival in Collinsville, Illinois, created to raise awareness for the herb in an area where much of the world's supply is grown.

 Ditch These Too!
Ranch dressing (2 Tbsp)
145 calories, 15.4 g fat, 245 mg sodium

Table salt (1 tsp)
0 calories, 0 fat, 2,325 mg sodium

Mayonnaise (2 Tbsp)
115 calories, 9.8 g fat, 209 mg sodium

≫ FAST FACT

The sharp tang of horseradish comes from a compound known as isothiocyanate, which can clear sinuses in some people. As well as boasting sinus-clearing abilities, horseradish has also been used as a low-back pain reliever and even an aphrodisiac!

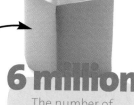

6 million

The number of gallons of horseradish prepared in the U.S. annually.

PICK IT

Nutritional Value

SERVING	2 Tbsp
CALORIES	65
FAT	0 g
CARBS	4.5 g
FIBER	0 g
SUGAR	4.5 g
SODIUM	45 mg
PROTEIN	11 g

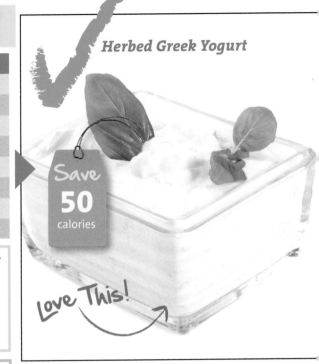

Herbed Greek Yogurt

Save
50
calories

Love This!

❯ QUICK & EASY
Add chopped cucumber to low-fat yogurt and use it as an accompaniment to cooked chicken or lamb.

❯❯ *FAST FACT*
Yogurt is a great bone builder, especially for young girls. A study published in the American Journal of Clinical Nutrition *noted that dairy foods such as yogurt may be better than a calcium supplement for bone-building.*

Give It a Try!

Nonfat greek style yogurt
90 calories, 0 fat, 7 g sugar

Wild Garden hummus dip
35 calories, 2 g fat, 70 mg sodium

Heinz cocktail sauce
35 calories, 2 g fat, 70 mg sodium

YES YOU CAN

Lose weight with a calcium-rich diet? You bet! Research on a group of women between the ages of 18 and 30 proves it – the women were put on either a low-calcium or a high-calcium diet for a year. After the year was over, the rate at which their bodies burned fat was analyzed – the fat burning was 20 times higher in the women who ate a high-calcium diet (1,000 – 1,400 mg per day).

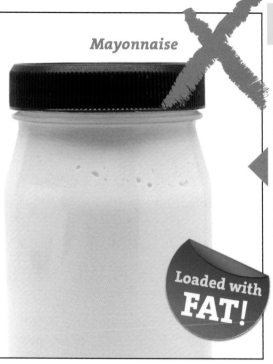

Mayonnaise

Loaded with FAT!

Nutritional Value	
SERVING	2 Tbsp
CALORIES	115
FAT	9.8 g
CARBS	7 g
FIBER	0 g
SUGAR	1.9 g
SODIUM	209 mg
PROTEIN	0.3 g

Say What?

EAT YOGURT and beat bad breath? It's true! Just 3.2 ounces of yogurt two times a day not only helps eliminate sulfide compounds that result in bad breath, but increasingly yogurt is found to help combat the risk of gingivitis and dental plaque.

61

Percentage more fat lost by women and men placed on a diet that included three daily portions of low-fat yogurt than others on a similar diet that did not include any yogurt at all. Not only did those in the yogurt group lose more fat, the loss was targeted around their waistlines .

Ditch These Too!

Hellmann's tartar sauce
160 calories, 14 g fat, 660 mg sodium

Tostitos creamy salsa
35 calories, 3 g fat, 150 mg sodium

Kraft Cheez Whiz dip
90 calories, 7 g fat, 440 mg sodium

The "healthy" bacteria **BONUS!**

in yogurt – the probiotic bacteria – may be able to shut down the *H. pylori* bacterium that's responsible for many ulcers. A recent study published in the *Journal of Nutrition* has also highlighted the "healthy" bacteria in yogurt for having positive effects on arthritis.

Your Top 15

PICK IT WINNERS!

So you want to get strong and lose weight? Here are 15 of the best ways to make small changes and get bigger results – it's easier than you think!

PICK IT ✓

Sweet Potatoes

Loaded with fiber and beta carotene, their complex carbohydrates are an excellent source of fuel for working out.

TIP: One medium sweet potato has 100 calories and is a source of iron, magnesium and vitamin B6.

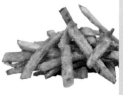

KICK IT ✗

White Potatoes

Not a great source of vitamins and minerals, nor do they provide long-lasting energy.

PICK IT ✓   KICK IT ✗

PICK IT		KICK IT	
Fresh or Frozen Fruit 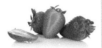	Try apples or berries for a high-fiber, low-calorie treat. **TIP: One large fresh apple with peel left on has five grams of fiber!**	*Canned Fruit* 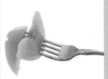	Loaded with sugar. No skin means a lot less fiber.
Oatmeal	High in fiber, helping to keep you full. **TIP: Only 83 calories for a half cup of cooked oats!**	*Store-Bought Granola, Including Bars*	Loaded with fat and sugar. **BETTER CHOICE: Low-fat varieties. Or better yet, make your own.**
Plain, Low-Fat Yogurt	A source of calcium and good bacteria. **TIP: Add fresh berries for a flavor boost.** **TIP: One 8-ounce serving of plain low-fat yogurt can have as much as 12 grams of protein.**	*Flavored Yogurt or Ice Cream* 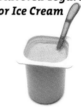	Available in fat-free versions, but can be loaded with sugar.
Broth-Based Soup CAUTION: *Watch the sodium level in prepared soup.*	A great way to get your veggies and satisfy hunger. **TIP: Cut the calories in half by choosing broth-based soups over cream-based.**	*Cream-Based Soup*	High in fat. **BETTER CHOICE: Make at home and substitute fat-free milk for cream.**
Baked or Grilled Fish 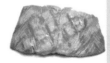	With muscle-building protein and essential fatty acids. **TIP: A three-ounce serving of baked wild Atlantic salmon has over five grams of healthy fats.**	*Fried, Breaded Fish* 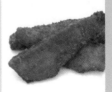	Saturated and trans fats.

PICK IT KICK IT

Baked Or Grilled Chicken Breast 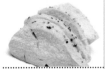	High in protein and low in fat. **TIP: Pass on the fat by choosing skinless breasts.**	***Fried, Breaded Chicken Strips***	Skip the breading and deep fryer.
Raw Unsalted Nuts and Seeds	Loaded with protein and healthy fats. Limit your daily serving to a third of a cup to keep the fat in check. **TIP: Make your own trail mix by adding some dried fruit.** **TIP: Choosing un-salted nuts can cut almost 200 mg of sodium per handful serving.**	***Salty Nuts, Potato Chips and Pretzels*** 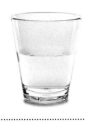	Salt and saturated fat.
Water	Keeps you hydrated. Be sure to drink at least eight 8-ounce glasses each day **TIP: Too boring? Add a splash of lemon or lime juice.** NO CALORIES!	***Alcohol and Soda*** 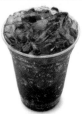	Sugar and booze are very dehydrating. FACT: **One can of soda = approximately 10 teaspoons of sugar.**
Dark Green Veggies 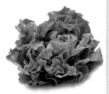	Provides vitamin A, vitamin C and calcium. **TIP: One cup of spinach has only seven calories.**	***Iceberg Lettuce*** 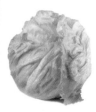	Low in vitamins and minerals. Try a dark green leafy lettuce in your salad. **TIP: When dining out, ask for dressing on the side and watch those top-pings!**

PICK IT ✓ KICK IT ✗

Low-Fat Milk 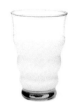	High in calcium and vitamin D. **TIP: A great addition to any smoothie or bowl of oatmeal.** **TIP: Choose fortified low-fat milk to get extra vitamin D in your diet.**	**High-Fat Milk** 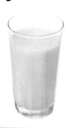	Higher in calories, not just fat.
Olive Oil, Fish Oil, Vegetable Oil 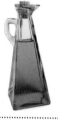	Use sparingly when cooking or making salad dressings to enhance flavor. Heart-healthy, but keep an eye on your portion. **TIP: One teaspoon of olive oil has 40 calories.**	**Butter, Vegetable Shortening, Margarine** 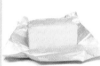	Skip these fats – they're loaded with saturated and trans fats.
Fruit Juice	A great substitute when fresh fruit isn't an option. Just be careful not to drink too many calories. **TIP: One cup of orange juice contains 100 percent of the RDA for vitamin C.**	**Fruit Drink**	Sugar, calories and very little fruit.
Whole Grains (Bread, Pasta, Rice and Flour)	Full of fiber, vitamins and minerals. **TIP: A slice of whole wheat bread has 100 calories and four grams of protein.**	**White, Refined Grains** 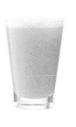	Stripped of fiber and nutrients, these provide short-lived energy.
Egg Whites	A fat-free protein.	**Egg Yolks**	Contain most of the egg's fat and cholesterol.

PICK IT

Nutritional Value

SERVING	30 g
CALORIES	130
FAT	3 g
CARBS	22 g
FIBER	2 g
SUGAR	3 g
SODIUM	160 mg
PROTEIN	3 g

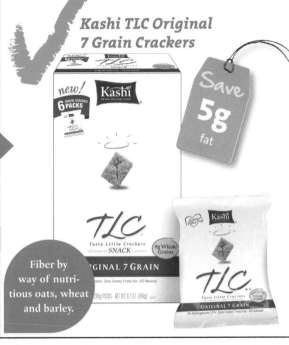

Kashi TLC Original 7 Grain Crackers

Save **5g** fat

Fiber by way of nutritious oats, wheat and barley.

BONUS!

Kashi
crackers are not only lower in sodium, they contain sea salt, which is much more mineral-dense than table salt.

TIP Better all round, Kashi crackers are higher in fiber and lower in sodium. Better yet? They don't have any saturated or trans fats at all!

Give It a Try!

Triscuits
120 calories, 4.5 g fat, 180 mg sodium

Ryvita crispbread
35 calories, 0 fat, 20 mg sodium

Vinta crackers
70 calories, 3 g fat, 110 mg sodium

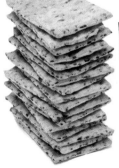

YES YOU CAN

Don't skip snacks. Research on gymnasts — some of the leanest athletes around — found that those who ate frequent, small meals and snacks had a lower body fat percentage than those who went longer without eating.

230

KICK IT

Ritz Crackers

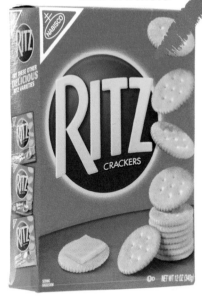

Nutritional Value	
SERVING	32 g
CALORIES	160
FAT	8 g
CARBS	20 g
FIBER	0 g
SUGAR	2 g
SODIUM	270 mg
PROTEIN	2 g

INSTANT MEAL COMBO

WHITE BEAN DIP

1 can white (cannelloni) beans

8 garlic gloves, roasted

2 Tbsp olive oil

2 Tbsp lemon juice

1. Rinse and drain beans.

2. Blend all ingredients until smooth.

3. Serve on Kashi or your favorite whole grain crackers.

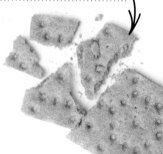

Ditch These Too!

Wheat Thins
140 calories, 6 g fat, 260 mg sodium

Cheez-It baked snack crackers
150 calories, 8 g fat, 250 mg sodium

Vegetable Thins
150 calories, 7 g fat, 330 mg sodium

Say What?

FIBER itself is nothing but carbohydrates that cannot be digested, which means that eating high-fiber products will help to stave off hunger for long periods of time.

PICK IT

Nutritional Value	
SERVING	20 oz
CALORIES	0
FAT	0 g
CARBS	0 g
FIBER	0 g
SUGAR	0 g
SODIUM	0 mg
PROTEIN	0 g

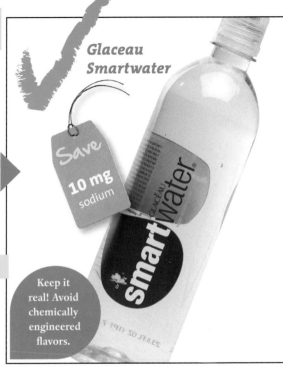

Glaceau Smartwater

Save 10 mg sodium

Keep it real! Avoid chemically engineered flavors.

BONUS!

Electrolye-rich

Glaceau Smartwater replaces important minerals lost after an intense workout – without the sugary, calorie-laden stuff found in common sports drinks.

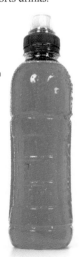

Give It a Try!

Lipton diet green tea with citrus (1 cup)
0 calories, 0 fat, 70 mg sodium

Low-sodium V8 vegetable juice (1 cup)
50 calories, 0 fat, 140 mg sodium

Orange juice (1 cup)
112 calories, 0.5 g fat, 2 mg sodium

Say What?

THE NEW YORK TIMES recently reported that some food companies use ambiguous wording on packaging to suggest that their products are healthier than they really are. Examine nutrition labels carefully and beware of false marketing claims.

KICK IT

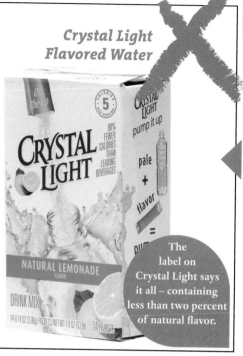

Crystal Light Flavored Water

The label on Crystal Light says it all – containing less than two percent of natural flavor.

Nutritional Value	
SERVING	2 g mixed in 8 fl oz water
CALORIES	5
FAT	0 g
CARBS	0 g
FIBER	0 g
SUGAR	0 g
SODIUM	10 mg
PROTEIN	0 g

TIP Keep an eye out for ingredients that sound like candy – citric acid, acesulfame potassium (sweetener) and artificial color.

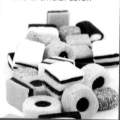

Ditch These Too!

Gatorade (20 oz)
123 calories, 0 fat, 493 mg sodium

Lemonade (1 cup)
99 calories, 0.1 g fat, 10 mg sodium

Ocean Spray cranberry juice (1 cup)
130 cups, 0 fat, 35 mg sodium

TIP Bored with drinking water? Looking for other ways to hydrate? Water is the best option, but there are other drinks and foods that can help provide the water your body needs. Stay away from drinks with added sugar and choose watery fruits and vegetables such as watermelon, tomatoes and lettuce.

Try This

If you're drinking coffee, tea or caffeinated soda, sip an extra glass of water for every mug you drink. Other beverages, such as juice and decaffeinated teas, can also add up. Drink one glass of water for each.

PICK IT

Nutritional Value	
SERVING	1 clove
CALORIES	4
FAT	0 g
CARBS	1 g
FIBER	0.1 g
SUGAR	0 g
SODIUM	1 mg
PROTEIN	0.2 g

Say What?

GARLIC IS an excellent source of manganese and vitamins B6 and C, and a good source of selenium. It also has the potential to keep your heart happy — it can positively affect everything from blood pressure to the risk of heart disease or stroke.

250 million

Number of pounds of garlic produced in California every year.

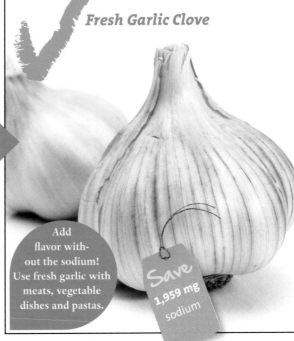

Fresh Garlic Clove

Add flavor without the sodium! Use fresh garlic with meats, vegetable dishes and pastas.

Save 1,959 mg sodium

Give It a Try!

Pesto (2 tsp)
45 calories, 4.5 g fat, 95 mg sodium

Tapenade
40 calories, 4 g fat, 290 mg sodium

Garlic mixed with low-fat yogurt and dill
77 calories, 0 fat, 87 sodium

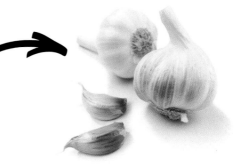

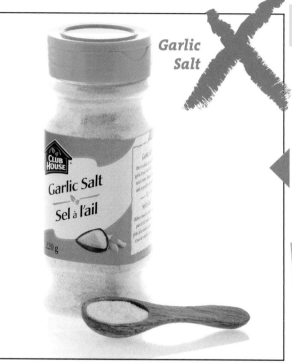

Garlic Salt

KICK IT

Nutritional Value	
SERVING	1 tsp
CALORIES	0
FAT	0 g
CARBS	0 g
FIBER	0 g
SUGAR	0 g
SODIUM	1,960 mg
PROTEIN	0 g

YES YOU CAN

Eat garlic and still have friends! Simply eat a sprig of parsley along with your meal and you will reduce the garlic smell on your breath. Or, try a lemon!

Ditch These Too!

Alfredo (2 tsp)
64 calories, 6.7 g fat, 47 mg sodium

Garlic butter
100 calories, 11 g fat, 110 mg sodium

Sour cream and chives
246 calories, 24.2 g fat, 61 mg sodium

BONUS!

The most potent active constituent in garlic, allicin, has been shown not only to lower blood pressure (according to research on animals), but also may prevent weight gain, according to a study published in the *American Journal of Hypertension*.

Say What?

GARLIC IS used in cooking in almost every culture and country in the world. China produces 66 percent of the world's garlic — 13 billion pounds in 2002. Next are South Korea (five percent), India (five percent) and the U.S. (three percent).

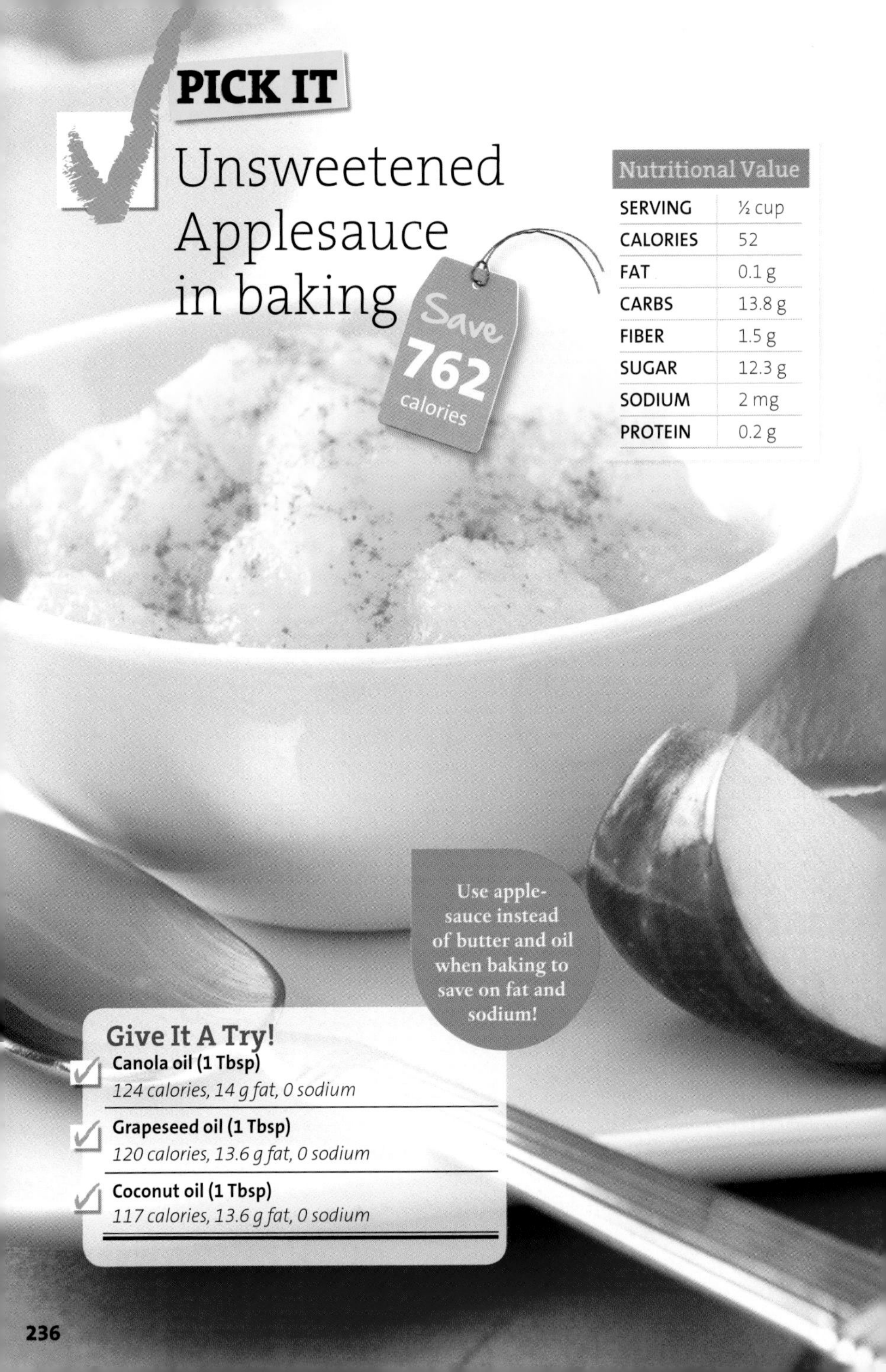

Unsweetened Applesauce in baking

Save
762
calories

Nutritional Value	
SERVING	½ cup
CALORIES	52
FAT	0.1 g
CARBS	13.8 g
FIBER	1.5 g
SUGAR	12.3 g
SODIUM	2 mg
PROTEIN	0.2 g

Use applesauce instead of butter and oil when baking to save on fat and sodium!

Give It A Try!

Canola oil (1 Tbsp)
124 calories, 14 g fat, 0 sodium

Grapeseed oil (1 Tbsp)
120 calories, 13.6 g fat, 0 sodium

Coconut oil (1 Tbsp)
117 calories, 13.6 g fat, 0 sodium

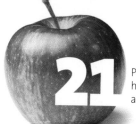

APPLESAUCE HAS NATURAL SUGARS!

21

Percentage less likelihood of having excess belly fat if you make apples a regular part of your diet.

QUICK & EASY

Add a tablespoon of natural peanut butter or ten nuts to your unsweetened applesauce for a great mid-morning or afternoon snack.

BONUS!

Using unsweetened applesauce in your baking is a sure way to avoid the dryness that often accompanies low-fat baked goods.

YES YOU CAN

Get long-lasting energy. The glycemic index is a measure of how quickly insulin is released after eating a food high in carbohydrates. A result above 70 is considered high and will put you on an energy roller coaster. Apples score low at 39, meaning steady energy for you.

The soluble fiber in apples can help reduce your cholesterol.

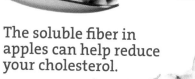

SAY WHAT? With four grams of fiber and just 80 calories, a small apple will fill you up and help you become slimmer. People currently enrolled in a large long-term weight-loss trial known as the Calerie Study, which is investigating whether calorie restriction can extend lifespan, have been getting thinner throughout the study. Their slimming strategy: eat an apple every day. And a recent study published in *Appetite* found that people who ate three apples a day versus three pears or three cookies lost about two pounds after ten weeks.

KICK IT

Oil or Butter in Baking

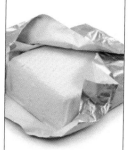

Nutritional Value

SERVING	½ cup
CALORIES	814
FAT	92 g
CARBS	0.1 g
FIBER	0 g
SUGAR	0.1 g
SODIUM	654 mg
PROTEIN	1 g

Ditch These Too!

Margarine (1 Tbsp)
*101 calories,
11.4 g fat,
93 mg sodium*

Lard (1 Tbsp)
*120 calories,
13 g fat,
0 sodium*

Vegetable shortening (1 Tbsp)
*115 calories,
12.8 g fat, 0 sodium*

PICK IT

Say What?

LEMONS, like other vitamin C-rich fruits, were highly prized during the California Gold Rush in the mid-19th century, since they were used to protect against scurvy.

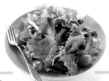

❯ QUICK & EASY

Mix up an easy, refreshing dressing for your next salad: mix lemon juice with olive or flax oil, freshly crushed garlic and pepper, or simply drizzle the juice of a lemon over greens (perfect for a workday lunch!).

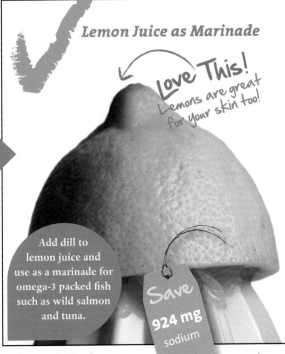

Lemon Juice as Marinade

Love This!
Lemons are great for your skin too!

Add dill to lemon juice and use as a marinade for omega-3 packed fish such as wild salmon and tuna.

Save 924 mg sodium

Give It a Try!

Low-sodium chicken broth (1 cup)
25 calories, 0.5 g fat, 140 mg sodium

Balsamic vinegar
15 calories, 0 g fat, 0 sodium

Pesto sauce (2 Tbsp)
95 calories, 9 g fat, 180 mg sodium

❯❯ FAST FACT

Lemons are loaded with Vitamin C, a great immune booster and anti-inflammatory.

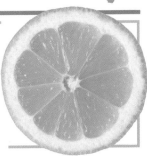

BBQ Sauce Marinade

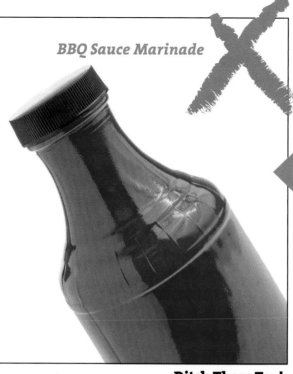

KICK IT

Nutritional Value	
SERVING	2 Tbsp
CALORIES	85
FAT	2 g
CARBS	14.5 g
FIBER	1.4 g
SUGAR	4.4 g
SODIUM	924 mg
PROTEIN	2 g

TIP Believe it or not, the tartness of a lemon makes for a great salt substitute – cut some wedges, and serve with any meal and hide the salt shaker in the cupboard

Ditch These Too!

Litehouse honey dijon marinade (2 Tbsp)
80 calories, 7 g fat, 280 mg sodium

Creamy garlic dressing (2 Tbsp)
120 calories, 13 g fat, 300 mg sodium

Clubhouse Greek marinade (1 serving)
98 calories, 0.4 g fat, 1,895 mg sodium

BONUS!

Place fresh lemon slices underneath fish just before you cook it. Add a bit of dill and you've got a tasty, low-fat, protein-packed meal!

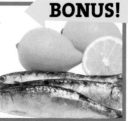

45

Percentage of the RDI for vitamin C contained in just a quarter cup of lemon juice.

PICK IT

Nutritional Value

SERVING	½ cup
CALORIES	100
FAT	1 g
CARBS	15.5 g
FIBER	7.5 g
SUGAR	1.5 g
SODIUM	340 mg
PROTEIN	6.5 g

▶ QUICK & EASY

In a small bowl, mix together black beans, guacamole, chopped tomatoes, diced onions and cilantro for a simple, tasty dip. (Go easy on the guacamole!)

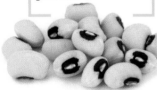

EVEN BETTER

Beans add a healthy dose of soluble and insoluble fiber, folic acid, protein and natural plant sterols that may help lower cholesterol, says Beth Thayer, M.S., R.D., of Detroit, a spokesperson for the American Dietetic Association.

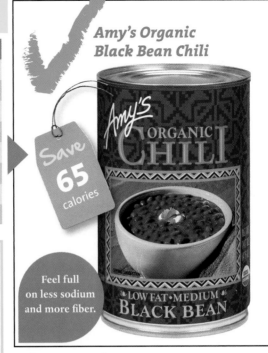

Amy's Organic Black Bean Chili

Save **65** calories

Feel full on less sodium and more fiber.

LOW FAT • MEDIUM
BLACK BEAN

Give It a Try!

Falafel
57 calories, 3 g fat, 50 mg sodium

Fried tofu (1 piece)
35 calories, 2.6 g fat, 2 mg sodium

Health Valley black bean soup (1 cup)
100 calories, 0 fat, 320 mg sodium

YES YOU CAN

Boost your nutrients and get a tasty meal that weighs in at only 100 calories. Chili is a nutritious meal any time of year, but you'll especially appreciate it during cold weather. In one dish, you get some of the best vitamins and minerals as well as fiber. Fiber is an important part of any fat-loss diet.

KICK IT

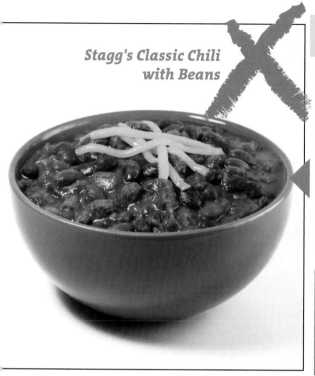

Stagg's Classic Chili with Beans

Nutritional Value	
SERVING	½ cup
CALORIES	165
FAT	8.5 g
CARBS	14 g
FIBER	2.5 g
SUGAR	3.5 g
SODIUM	410 mg
PROTEIN	8.5 g

BONUS!

Serve a cup of chili over brown rice or whole grain pasta, and you'll increase fiber, B vitamins and good carbs for energy.

Ditch These Too!

Meat lasagna (1 cup)
290 calories, 10 g fat, 490 mg sodium

Quiche Lorraine (1 serving)
419 calories, 28 g fat, 643 mg sodium

Thai fried noodles (1 serving)
367 calories, 18 g fat, 303 mg sodium

TIP Make a big pot of chili on the weekend and freeze leftovers in meal-sized containers for quick suppers later.

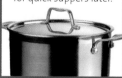

Say What?

ORIGINALLY A STAPLE on cattle drives in the Southwest, basic chili combines well-seasoned and well-cooked meat with chili peppers. You'll find regional variations of it across the country – from vegetarian to meat only and served in bowls, in buns and over hot dogs. In some places, the best way to enjoy chili is to serve it over spaghetti.

29.5

Percentage of the recommended daily value of fiber contained in just one cup of black beans.

PICK IT

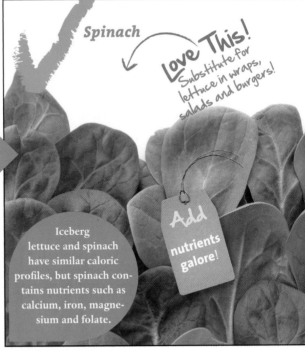

Spinach

Love This! Substitute for lettuce in wraps, salads and burgers!

Add nutrients galore!

Nutritional Value	
SERVING	1 cup
CALORIES	7
FAT	0.1 g
CARBS	1.1 g
FIBER	0.7 g
SUGAR	0.1 g
SODIUM	24 mg
PROTEIN	0.9 g

TIP When shopping for leafy greens, stick to this simple, easy-to-remember rule: the darker the greens, the more nutrient-rich and the better choice!

Iceberg lettuce and spinach have similar caloric profiles, but spinach contains nutrients such as calcium, iron, magnesium and folate.

MAKE IT BETTER

Keep it all in the family and try some Swiss chard. Dark green vegetables are a staple of any clean diet and Swiss chard is one of the very best. A one-cup serving of cooked chard provides 214 percent of your daily vitamin A, over 700 percent of your vitamin K and is a good source of vitamin C, iron, calcium, vitamin E and magnesium ... all in a 35-calorie package.

Give It a Try!

Spinach salad, no dressing (1 cup)
81 calories, 2 g fat, 133 mg sodium

Roasted potatoes (½ cup)
131 calories, 4 g fat, 37 mg sodium

Steamed broccoli (½ cup)
27 calories, 0.3 g fat, 32 mg sodium

≫ FAST FACT

California is the top spinach-producing state in the U.S. It's responsible for three-quarters of all spinach production. Other states that grow and supply spinach are New Jersey, Arizona, Arkansas, Texas and Colorado.

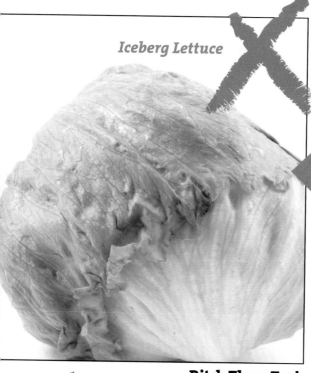

Iceberg Lettuce

KICK IT

Nutritional Value	
SERVING	1 cup
CALORIES	8
FAT	0.1 g
CARBS	1.7 g
FIBER	0.7 g
SUGAR	1 g
SODIUM	6 mg
PROTEIN	0.5 g

BONUS!

Spinach is a good choice for all kinds of reasons – at least 13 of them! There are at least 13 compounds in spinach that are antioxidants and act as anti-cancer agents.

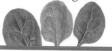

Ditch These Too!

Creamy coleslaw (½ cup)
190 calories, 20 g fat, 125 mg sodium

Potato salad (½ cup)
217 calories, 12 g fat, 380 mg sodium

Broccoli bacon salad (½ cup)
324 calories, 31.6 g fat, 186 mg sodium

Say What?

SPINACH CONTAINS a host of nutrients including beta-carotene, vitamin C and vitamin K, all of which have anti-inflammatory properties. But there's more – the magnesium and riboflavin in spinach may also help if you suffer from migraines.

18

Number of milligrams of iron women aged 19 to 50 need daily to keep their energy levels peaked, according to the National Institutes of Health. (Spinach is a great source!)

PICK IT

Nutritional Value	
SERVING	½ cup
CALORIES	77
FAT	2 g
CARBS	8.6 g
FIBER	0 g
SUGAR	8.6 g
SODIUM	86 mg
PROTEIN	6.4 g

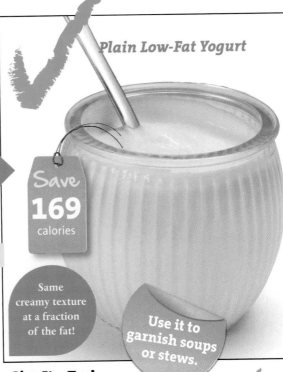

Plain Low-Fat Yogurt

Save
169
calories

Same creamy texture at a fraction of the fat!

Use it to garnish soups or stews.

BONUS!

Yogurt

contains bone-building calcium and it's also a good staple for your fat loss – a higher calcium intake is associated with lower body-fat levels, partly thanks to its high concentration of the amino acid leucine.

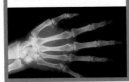

Give It a Try!

Calcium-enriched orange juice (1 cup)
120 calories, 0 fat, 10 mg sodium ✓

Low-fat cottage cheese (1 cup)
163 calories, 2.3 g fat, 918 mg sodium ✓

Calcium-fortified milk (1 cup)
80 calories, 0 fat, 125 mg sodium ✓

Say What?

PROBIOTICS, aka "good bacteria" make yogurt a nutritional powerhouse. They prevent and treat gastrointestinal problems such as constipation, diarrhea, bloating and gas – factors that may occur at the onset of starting your new clean diet. Look for the words "Lactobacillus" and "Bifidobacterium" on yogurt labels, as these are the specific strains research shows are most beneficial to active people.

Sour Cream

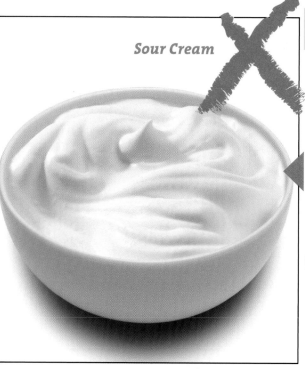

KICK IT

Nutritional Value	
SERVING	½ cup
CALORIES	246
FAT	24.2 g
CARBS	4.9 g
FIBER	0 g
SUGAR	0.2 g
SODIUM	61 mg
PROTEIN	3.6 g

YES YOU CAN Build stronger bones. To prevent osteoporosis and keep your bones healthy, you should get a bone mineral density test (BMD), do weight-bearing exercises and get 1,000 mg of calcium a day in addition to 500 mg of magnesium and 400 IU of vitamin D. These things will work hand in hand to improve bone density.

Ditch These Too!
French onion dip (2 Tbsp)
60 calories, 5 g fat, 220 mg sodium

Sweet and sour sauce (2 Tbsp)
60 calories, 0 fat, 130 mg sodium

Fritos bean dip (2 Tbsp)
40 calories, 1 g fat, 190 mg sodium

YES YOU CAN Have a healthier body just by eating the right foods. Plain, low-fat yogurt is a good source of energy-boosting vitamins B5 and B12, along with zinc and a trace mineral that helps detoxify your body, called molybdenum.

> ## QUICK & EASY
Mix
- 8 oz yogurt
- 1 tsp parsley
- 1 tsp cilantro
- 1 tsp onion, chopped
- ½ tsp celery salt.
Chill in the fridge for one hour. Use as a dip for carrots, celery and bell peppers.

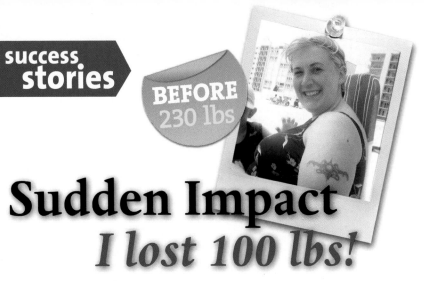

BEFORE
230 lbs

Sudden Impact
I lost 100 lbs!

A life-changing accident gave Miranda Henderson the determination she needed to get strong and reach her fat-loss goals. BY JUDI KETTELER

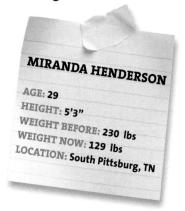

MIRANDA HENDERSON

AGE: 29
HEIGHT: 5'3"
WEIGHT BEFORE: 230 lbs
WEIGHT NOW: 129 lbs
LOCATION: South Pittsburg, TN

Waking up in the hospital after a car accident, Miranda Henderson had no idea she just spent an entire month in a coma. She had undergone heart surgery and her lungs weren't functioning properly. As she came to, she had no strength and her motor skills were gone. She couldn't even hold a Popsicle in her hands.

STARTING OVER

Before the accident, Miranda had been on the way to a lifestyle change. Growing up in the heart of deep-fried Southern culture, she weighed 230 lbs at her heaviest and was also a chain-smoker. "I knew that I was heading down the wrong road, and I was unhappy with myself and my choices," she says. Before the accident she had started to educate herself about health and fitness, and she had started to lose weight by walking and watching her food portions, but lacked the focus and strong drive to reach her goals. Now, in the hospital, she would have to re-learn how to do everything from walking to tying her shoes. But she was determined to succeed. "I told myself: 'My body has been through this awful trauma. It deserves to be treated healthy,'" she says.

BALANCED PLAN

Once recovered, Miranda realized that she needed a real plan – one that incorporated weight training and cardio, and involved a healthy diet that would help her build strength and not just lose weight. "When I got to the gym the first time, I was lost," she says. The owner walked her through a routine, but it left her so sore the next day that she could barely sit down. Not wanting to quit before she had truly begun, Miranda backed off a little. She focused on mastering some classic exercises such as triceps kickbacks, biceps curls, leg extensions (on the machine), and squats and lunges (with and without weights). She also fell in love with her kickboxing DVD, started spinning classes and learned new moves by reading *Oxygen*.

Discovering clean eating completed the picture for Miranda. "When I read *The Eat-Clean Diet*, by Tosca Reno, I hadn't heard of half the stuff in there. I remember thinking: 'What in the world is flaxseed?'" she says. She was hesitant to start, but tried the two-week meal plan. Once she got familiar with the foods, she found that she enjoyed eating clean. "I love the simplicity of it and the idea that you just keep things as natural as you can." Still, friends and family found it difficult to understand her new habits. "When you don't want to eat something someone has made for you because it's fried, for example, it hurts their feelings," she says. But Miranda continued on, finally reaching a healthy weight of 129 lbs.

NEW CONFIDENCE

Now, Miranda sees that the benefits of her fit lifestyle stretch beyond fat loss. "Since I've started taking care of myself, I have become a happy, confident woman," she says. Miranda hopes to start competing in fitness, and it will take more than some criticism or a set of sizzling deep fryers to stop her. "You have to keep your eyes on the prize," she says.

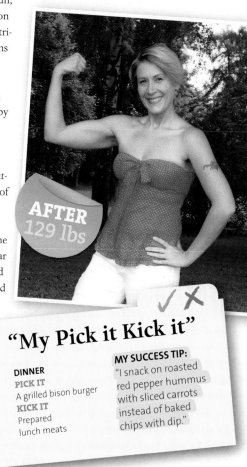

AFTER
129 lbs

"My Pick it Kick it"

DINNER
PICK IT
A grilled bison burger
KICK IT
Prepared lunch meats

MY SUCCESS TIP:
"I snack on roasted red pepper hummus with sliced carrots instead of baked chips with dip."

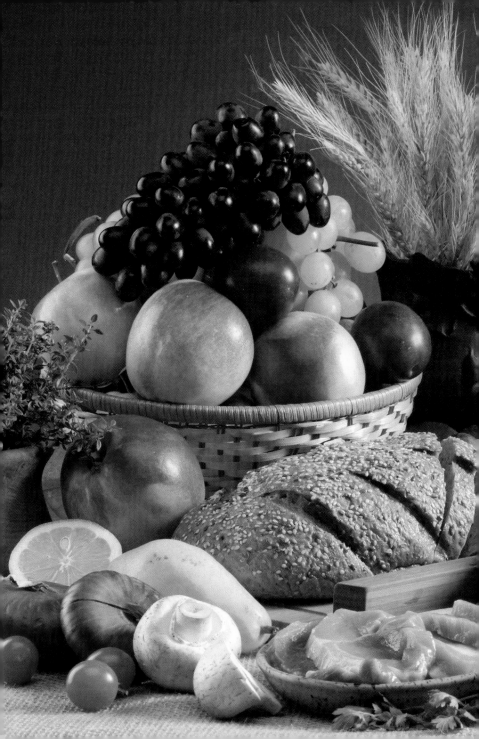

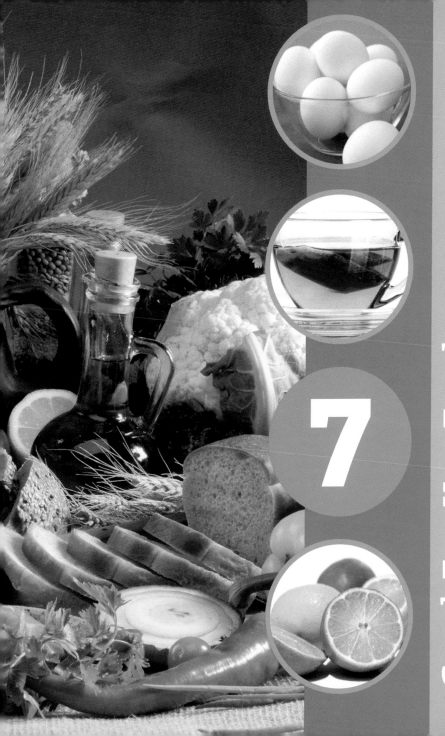

7

Good-For-You Foods

EAT BETTER FEEL BETTER!

Want to be at your best?
Start with a smarter diet and choose good-for-you foods that bolster your immune system (to ward off colds and flu), keep your body energized (to help you stay fit and lean) and let you sleep better. What more could you want?

I gave up two "staples" in my kitchen many years ago that made all the difference in my energy levels and weight management: soda pop and the salt shaker. Get rid of both (or one to start) and trust me, you'll see the difference in many ways – from jeans that start to fit to a better night's sleep.

Soda pop is one of the cheapest beverages on the market, but researchers and health authorities are becoming concerned with just how popular it's becoming. Today, Americans drink 200 percent more soda pop than we did in the late 1970s, which is 200 percent more calories, too. With the average person in the U.S. drinking 50 gallons of soda every year – that's a ton of sugar!

Health authorities have already linked the abundance of salt in processed foods to many ailments and diseases, and the new culprit is soda because it's very high in sugar. In fact, you shouldn't be surprised to find yourself shelling out a special "sin" tax on soda, similar to those on tobacco, alcohol and gasoline. A handful of states have already imposed a tax on soda, including Arkansas, Tennessee, Virginia and Washington.

You'd be wise to swap out the salt and sugary soda in your diet. By doing so, you'll reduce your risk of developing one or more of the many health problems plaguing Americans.

And at the grocery store, you'll have more room in your cart for better food choices. Choosing nutrient-rich essentials during your next grocery run will help you stay energized all day and get you closer to meeting your fat-loss goals.

Certain vitamins and minerals may aid your efforts. "Consuming foods high in magnesium, for instance, can assist with weight loss because it contains fatigue-fighting chemicals," says Amy Jamieson-Petonic, RD, a spokesperson for the American Dietetic Association and manager at The Cleveland Clinic. Other nutrients that keep you lean are calcium, potassium and fiber.

Snacking on an apple (with the peel still intact) provides you with enough dietary fiber to help maintain energy levels throughout a workout, says Jamieson-Petonic. And don't forget to pick up some lean beef and chickpeas when you're in the grocery store, too. "Foods containing iron will enhance your energy by delivering oxygen to your cells," she says.

Choosing more good-for-you foods (they appear as the "picks"), ditch the ones that are the "kick" and you'll be well on your way to getting the body you want.

A good night's sleep is also vital for fat loss. To be at your best, you need rest – it's that simple. Yet half of all Americans say they don't sleep well five nights a week. (It's little wonder that sleep aid companies are doing so well!) Try to get seven to eight hours of sleep every night – recent studies show that anything less may cause you to pack on the pounds. "Sleep deprivation can interfere with ghrelin and leptin, two hormones that play a major role in appetite regulation," says Sarah Meyers, a registered dietitian at the University of Michigan Cardiovascular Center. Swap out caffeine for a soothing warm cup of low-fat milk, try not to eat at least three hours before crawling into bed and stay away from your laptop, too. The glare from the screen mimics sunlight and can trick your brain into thinking it's daytime.

Finally, while enjoying more good-for-you foods, you'll also need to modify your liquid needs. You may often reach for something to eat when you aren't really hungry – you're actually thirsty. And, if you're 60 years old or older, your ability to recognize thirst will start to drop, which means that it's more important than ever to keep water, and not soda, at hand. "Every cell in your body needs water and if you are dehydrated, it's more difficult to burn fat," says Jamieson-Petonic. Instead of sipping a soda, which is nutrient-bereft, curb your thirst with a refreshing glass of water or calcium-rich low-fat milk.

In the next pages you'll find an amazing array of information on what to choose to make you look and feel better. It's all about making smarter choice and ultimately, the choice is yours. Choose wisely and you'll be able to lose weight more easily, have more energy for your busy day and actually go to sleep when your head hits the pillow at night.

SHAKE YOUR SALT HABIT

Even if you've given up the salt shaker for years, you could still be getting more heart-damaging sodium in your diet than you think. Find out how you can eat clean without sacrificing taste – while keeping your heart and waistline in shape.

Bonus: 3 tasty low-sodium recipes!

BY JILL MORAN | PHOTOGRAPHY PETER CHOU

As a clean eater, you may think that you don't need to watch your sodium intake. But busy exercise-loving women like you are notorious convenience eaters, picking up seemingly healthy foods at the supermarket – such as low-fat frozen dinners, protein bars, cereals and low-fat cottage cheese – to fuel their active lifestyles. While these foods appear to be the better buy nutritionally, they can contain significant amounts of salt. One cup of cottage cheese, for example, has a whopping 918 mg of sodium! How can salt derail your fitness goals? Experts say the health risks go beyond the temporary belly pooch you get after eating a salty Mexican meal. "Excess salt damages cells and damaged cells don't function at their best. This means all bodily processes will suffer, including your metabolism and your ability to burn fat and repair muscle," says Lyssie Lakatos, RD, coauthor of *The Secret to Skinny: How Salt Makes You Fat* (Health Communications, Inc., 2009). Read on to discover the benefits of slashing salt.

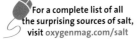
For a complete list of all the surprising sources of salt, visit oxygenmag.com/salt

Did you know?

According to the American Heart Association, the average American eats double the daily recommended amount of sodium (a little more than one teaspoon!).

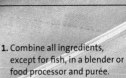

Jerk Fish

Ready in 1 ½ hours • Makes 4 servings

4 cloves garlic, roughly chopped
----
1 medium yellow onion, chopped
----
1 scotch bonnet (or habañero) pepper or 1 jalapeno pepper, seeded and roughly chopped
----
Juice of 1 lime
----
2 Tbsp olive oil
----
2 Tbsp 100% natural maple syrup
----
2 tsp thyme
----
2 tsp black pepper
----
2 tsp allspice
----
1 tsp cinnamon

½ tsp nutmeg
----
1 lb tilapia
----

1. Combine all ingredients, except for fish, in a blender or food processor and purée.

2. Place fish in a bowl and coat with purée. Let marinate for at least one hour or up to a day.

3. When ready to cook, spray a large skillet with nonstick spray over medium-high heat. Add fish and cook, about three to five minutes on each side. Serve with vegetables.

Nutrients per serving: Calories: 225, Total Fats: 10 g, Saturated Fat: 2 g, Trans Fat: 0 g, Cholesterol: 57 mg, Sodium: 61 mg, Total Carbohydrates: 13 g, Dietary Fiber: 1 g, Sugar: 9 g, Protein: 23 g, Iron: 1 mg

BYE-BYE, BLOAT!

"Eating too much sodium can cause you to retain fluid, which can increase your weight temporarily," says Jeannie Moloo, PhD, RD, spokesperson for the American Dietetic Association, coauthor of *The No-Salt, Lowest Sodium Cookbook* (St. Martin's Press, 2007). That's because salt is hydrophilic (water loving), which means that your body retains water to dilute the sodium concentration to a healthier level. As a result, you urinate less and this can lead to the dreaded belly bloat.

The best way to find out if you are consuming more than the recommended daily intake is to track the sodium content in your meals for a few days. Is your daily intake more than 2,300 mg? If so, try to reduce your intake to about 1,500 mg per day. Aim to:

• Eat fresh foods over their processed, packaged counterparts.

• Avoid foods that are cured, smoked and pickled – choose baked or grilled.

• Choose spices and herbs to add flavor to your meals in lieu of table salt. (See Flavor Boosters for a list of the best.)

• Choose sea salt over table salt. It has more muscle-relaxing magnesium than table salt and a truer, saltier taste, which helps you reduce the need to consume a lot of it.

• Snuff out sodium's many aliases on the ingredient list, such as monosodium glutamate (MSG), baking powder and baking soda.

... or follow our 3-Day Low-Sodium Meal Plan on page 257.

Herbed Lentils
Ready in 45 minutes • Makes 4 servings

1 Tbsp olive oil

2 carrots, diced

2 celery stalks, diced

1 medium yellow onion, diced

4 cloves garlic, diced

1 cup dried lentils, rinsed and picked through

2 sprigs fresh thyme, bruised*

1 stalk fresh rosemary, bruised

Water (about 2 cups)

2 tsp olive oil

Juice of ½ lemon

2 tsp red wine vinegar

*To bruise: gently roll and rub herbs in your hands.

1. Put oil in a medium pot. Add vegetables and garlic. Sauté over medium heat until softened.

2. Add lentils, thyme, rosemary and water. Bring to a boil, reduce heat to a simmer and cover. Cook until lentils are soft, about 25 minutes.

3. Remove thyme and rosemary sprigs and transfer lentils to a bowl. Add oil, lemon juice and vinegar and stir.

Pair with a complex carb, such as barley or quinoa, for a balanced meal.

Nutrients per serving: Calories: 165, Total Fats: 6 g, Saturated Fat: 1 g, Trans Fat: 0 g, Cholesterol: 0 mg, Sodium: 49 mg, Total Carbohydrates: 28 g, Dietary Fiber: 13 g, Sugar: 5 g, Protein: 11 g, Iron: 1 mg

RELIEVE YOUR HEART

It's important to keep in mind that salt is not the sole culprit of heart disease, which is the number one killer of women in America. A high-salt diet is often laden with fat and cholesterol, and it is this treacherous trio that works collectively to damage the ticker that keeps you going. Don't wait until your blood pressure creeps up to start paying attention to the salt in your foods, experts advise. Heart disease is no longer considered an older woman's disease. According to the Centers for Disease Control and Prevention, heart disease is the third leading cause of death among women 44 years of age and under. Reducing your salt intake now can prevent heart problems for you down the road. "Women who practice healthy lifestyle habits – such as exercising regularly and eating a balanced diet of lean protein, whole grains, fruits, vegetables and healthy fats – should also watch their sodium intake from processed fare to help prevent developing high blood pressure," Moloo says.

SLIM UP FOR GOOD

According to a growing body of evidence, salt contributes to the country's rising obesity rate because salty foods also tend to be high in other diet disasters, such as fat and sugar, which undeniably boost the taste of foods. "This is what can lead to overeating and cause weight gain for many people," Moloo says. Because glucose is the brain's food of choice and fat is an extremely rich source of calories, our bodies are evolutionarily primed to prefer foods that are high in both. However, because salt is essential to life, the body is driven to eat it above just about all else. That makes it extremely difficult to train a tongue that's accustomed to salty foods not to eat as much of them. Still, it can be done. In fact, in less than a month, you can retrain your taste buds to be more sensitive to salt while you decrease it from your diet.

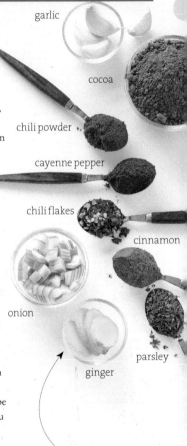

garlic

cocoa

chili powder

cayenne pepper

chili flakes

cinnamon

onion

parsley

ginger

Your salt stand-ins *flavor boosters*

One of the benefits of using herbs and spices and other fragrant foods in cooking instead of salt is that so many of them are what can be considered "functional foods." Try adding a few of these to your meals and benefit from their health-boosting effects.

TO IMPROVE YOUR...	TOSS IN SOME...
metabolism	chili powder, chili flakes, cayenne pepper, ginger
insulin sensitivity	cinnamon
blood flow	cocoa
immunity	garlic, onion
hormone balance	parsley

TURN FOR SOLUTIONS.

YOUR SODIUM SOLUTION

The clincher is that sodium is necessary for the proper functioning of your body (see 4 Reasons Why You Need Some Salt). But, the key is keeping intake low. You increase your risk of heart disease and weight gain when modern processed foods become the main part of your diet. The answer is to be vigilant and be aware of the sodium content in anything that comes packaged – especially those products that are marketed to you, the fit woman. When you slash the salt, your heart and belly will thank you for it.

Chicken Curry

Ready in 25 minutes • Makes 3 servings

1 Tbsp olive oil

1 onion, thinly sliced

4 cloves garlic, diced

2 tsp fresh ginger, grated

3 Tbsp curry powder

1/2 tsp cinnamon

1 tsp cumin

1 lb chicken breasts, cut into chunks

1 cup coconut milk

1/2 cup water

1/2 cup low-fat (2%) Greek yogurt

Juice of 1/2 lemon

1. Coat a large skillet with oil and place over medium heat.

2. Saute onions until softened, about two minutes, then add garlic, ginger, curry, cinnamon and cumin. Stir to combine. Add chicken and let sear, about two minutes.

3. Add coconut milk, water and yogurt, stir to coat and let simmer, stirring occasionally, until chicken is cooked through, about 20 minutes. Add lemon juice and stir to combine.

Nutrients per serving:
Calories: 327, Total Fats: 15 g, Saturated Fat: 9 g, Trans Fat: 0 g, Cholesterol: 90 mg, Sodium: 118 mg, Total Carbohydrates: 8 g, Dietary Fiber: 1 g, Sugar: 3 g, Protein: 40 g, Iron: 2 mg

The bulk of your salt intake comes from pre-packaged foods.

77%
from processed and prepared foods

12%
from natural sources

6%
added while eating

5%
added while cooking

SHAKE LESS, SLIM DOWN

The turmeric in curry powder is a potent inflammation fighter, and ginger can boost your metabolism to help burn fat.

3-DAY LOW-SODIUM MEAL PLAN

This meal plan supports a 130-pound woman.

DAY ONE:
WORKOUT DAY

DAILY TOTAL: Calories: 1,609, Protein(g): 143, Carbs(g): 215, Fat(g): 38, Sodium(mg): 1,413

BREAKFAST
2 whole large eggs
1 large egg white
1 cup oatmeal, cooked
1 cup strawberries, sliced

LUNCH
Turkey Wrap:
1 whole wheat tortilla
- - - - - - - - - - - - - - - -
4 oz reduced-sodium
  deli turkey breast
- - - - - - - - - - - - - - - -
½ cup romaine lettuce
- - - - - - - - - - - - - - - -
1 tomato, sliced

PREWORKOUT
7 oz reduced-fat (2%) Greek
  yogurt
2 Tbsp honey

POSTWORKOUT
1 scoop whey protein powder
10 oz fruit juice

DINNER
**CHICKEN CURRY
(SEE PAGE 256)**
½ cup brown rice, cooked
1 cup butternut squash
8 asparagus spears

DAY TWO:
WORKOUT DAY

DAILY TOTAL: Calories: 1,634, Protein(g): 140, Carbs(g) 163, Fat(g): 60, Sodium(mg): 1,092

BREAKFAST
*Cheese Scramble
Sandwich:*
2 large whole eggs
- - - - - - - - - - - - - - - -
1 large egg white
- - - - - - - - - - - - - - - -
2 oz low-fat cheddar cheese, grated
- - - - - - - - - - - - - - - -
1 whole wheat English muffin

LUNCH
Deli Salad:
**4 oz no-sodium-added
  deli roast beef**
- - - - - - - - - - - - - - - -
2 cups salad
- - - - - - - - - - - - - - - -
1 tomato, diced
- - - - - - - - - - - - - - - -
½ English cucumber, diced
- - - - - - - - - - - - - - - -
**1 Tbsp oil and vinegar salad
  dressing**
- - - - - - - - - - - - - - - -
¼ cup walnuts

PREWORKOUT
1 scoop whey protein powder
  mixed with water
1 medium banana

POSTWORKOUT
1 scoop whey protein powder
10 oz fruit juice

DINNER
JERK FISH (SEE PAGE 253)
1 large sweet potato
1 cup zucchini, sliced

DAY THREE:
REST DAY

DAILY TOTAL: Calories: 1,415, Protein(g): 131, Carbs(g): 107, Fat(g): 52, Sodium(mg): 1,282

BREAKFAST
2 whole large eggs
1 large egg white
1 cup oatmeal, cooked

MID-MORNING SNACK
8 oz low-fat (1%)
  no-sodium-added cottage
  cheese
1 medium peach

LUNCH
Tuna Pita:
**4 oz of canned water-
  packed albacore tuna, drained**
- - - - - - - - - - - - - - - -
1 Tbsp light mayonnaise
- - - - - - - - - - - - - - - -
½ cup spinach
- - - - - - - - - - - - - - - -
1 small whole wheat pita

AFTERNOON SNACK
2 stalks celery
2 Tbsp natural peanut butter

DINNER
4 oz chicken breast
**HERBED LENTILS
(SEE PAGE 254)**
2 cups spinach or other greens
1 Tbsp oil and vinegar salad
  dressing

4 REASONS WHY YOU NEED (SOME) SALT

1. **You sweat.** After a good bout of cardio (more than an hour), sodium replenishes the electrolytes you lose when you sweat, reducing your risk of losing neuromuscular function, which can lead to dizzy spells and, at worst, hyponatremia.

2. **You lift weights.** Sodium's function in nerve impulse transmission and muscular contraction helps to support your training.

3. **You want muscle.** Research shows that salt may improve protein synthesis by pushing creatine into the muscle cells.

4. **You need to function.** Sodium is an essential mineral (don't forget that!). Its role in nerve impulse transmission enables cells to send messages back and forth between themselves so you can think, see and perform everyday tasks.

PICK IT

Nutritional Value	
SERVING	1 tsp
CALORIES	0
FAT	0 g
CARBS	0 g
FIBER	0 g
SUGAR	0 g
SODIUM	0 mg
PROTEIN	0 g

 FAST FACT

One tablespoon of soy sauce delivers nearly 40 percent of your allowable daily quota of sodium.

90

Percentage of food allergies associated with only eight types of food, soy sauce being among them, according to the CDC. If you're allergic to soy sauce, some of the symptoms may include skin conditions such as itching and eczema, nasal congestion, canker sores, shortness of breath, fatigue and weakness.

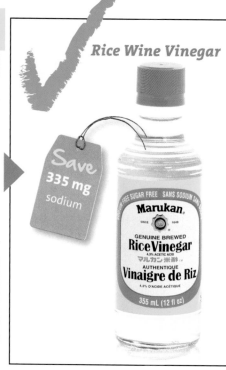

Rice Wine Vinegar

Save 335 mg sodium

Marukan
SINCE 1649
GENUINE BREWED
RiceVinegar
4.3% ACETIC ACID
マルカン米酢
AUTHENTIQUE
Vinaigre de Riz
4.3% D'ACIDE ACÉTIQUE
355 mL (12 fl oz)

Give It a Try!

Balsamic vinegar (1 Tbsp)
10 calories, 0 fat, 0 sodium ✓

Fat-free raspberry vinaigrette (1.5 oz)
50 calories, 0 fat, 320 mg sodium ✓

White wine vinegar (1 Tbsp)
0 calories, 0 fat, 0 sodium ✓

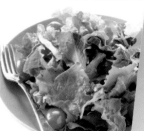

Try This

Rice wine vinegar is said to be a perfect complement for sweet sauces. And because of its light taste, you can also add it to your salads or drizzle it on steamed veggies.

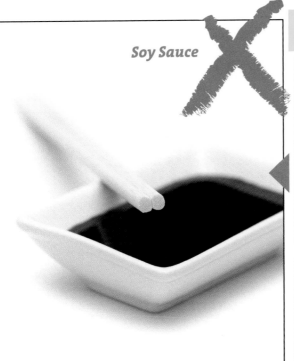

Soy Sauce

KICK IT

Nutritional Value	
SERVING	1 tsp
CALORIES	4
FAT	0 g
CARBS	0.3 g
FIBER	0 g
SUGAR	0.1 g
SODIUM	335 mg
PROTEIN	0.6 g

 FAST FACT

Used widely in China, Japan, Korea and Vietnam, rice wine vinegar is made from fermented rice wine and can be purchased either seasoned or un-seasoned (with garlic, red pepper flakes, oregano, blueberry, apricot or tarragon, among other options). It is much less acidic and milder than distilled western varieties of vinegar.

Ditch These Too!

 Ranch dressing (1 Tbsp)
74 calories, 7.8 g fat, 143.5 mg sodium

 Honey mustard dressing (1 Tbsp)
65 calories, 5.5 g fat, 105 mg sodium

 Teriyaki marinade (1 Tbsp)
15 calories, 0 fat, 610 mg sodium

Say What?

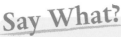

THREE TABLESPOONS of soy sauce – much less that what many people eat with their sushi meal – will put you beyond your daily threshold limit for sodium. The only way to offset this excessively high intake is to avoid all other salt-containing products that day, which is a virtually impossible goal. Exceed your sodium limit habitually, and, according to a very recent study, you'll significantly increase your risk for stroke and cardiovascular disease.

PICK IT

Nutritional Value

SERVING	1 oz
CALORIES	98
FAT	0.6 g
CARBS	23.1 g
FIBER	3.5 g
SUGAR	0 g
SODIUM	0 mg
PROTEIN	3.5 g

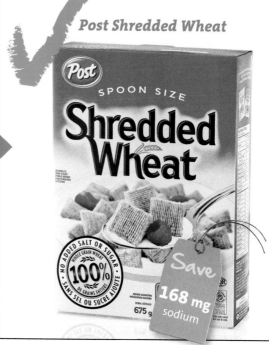

Post Shredded Wheat

Save **168 mg** sodium

IDEAL BREAKFAST

Most nutritionists agree that a healthy breakfast improves metabolism (which helps you manage your weight), controls hunger pangs later in the day (reducing binge eating), and provides sustained energy. Your breakfast should include some form of protein in addition to complex carbohydrates.

80

Percentage of the population not eating the recommended levels of whole grains.

Give It a Try!

Weetabix (1 cup)
213 calories, 2 g fat, 6 g fiber

Grape Nuts (½ cup)
208 calories, 1 g fat, 5 g fiber

Wheat Chex (¾ cup)
169 calories, 1 g fat, 5 g fiber

Say What?

WHEN A GRAIN IS REFINED, the bran and germ are removed, and along with them a significant amount of important nutrients. Enriching the resulting flour with certain vitamins and minerals does not make up for the deficits created by refining. Stick to whole grains, which contain a wealth of micronutrients along with fiber and heart-healthy fats.

Kellogg's Raisin Bran

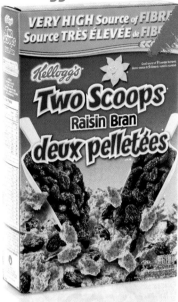

Nutritional Value	
SERVING	1 oz
CALORIES	91
FAT	0.7 g
CARBS	21.6 g
FIBER	3.4 g
SUGAR	9.1 g
SODIUM	168 mg
PROTEIN	2.4 g

Try This

In need of a quick energy fix? Crush three Spoon Size Shredded Wheat biscuits and mix them with a third cup of unsweetened applesauce, let the cereal soften (a couple of minutes) and then eat. The applesauce will give you a near-instant energy spike while the complex nature of the shredded wheat will prevent an energy sag later on.

Ditch These Too!

 Kellogg's Corn Flakes (1 cup)
101 calories, 0.2 g fat, 0.7 g fiber

 Apple Cinnamon Cheerios (1 cup)
120 calories, 2 g fat, 1 g fiber

 Post Golden Crisp (¾ cup)
107 calories, 0 fat, 0 fiber

1893

The year lawyer and businessman Henry Drushel Perky invented Shredded Wheat to help him control heartburn. He called his invention "little whole wheat mattresses."

≫ FAST FACT

The word "cereal" has its roots in the name "Ceres," not surprisingly the Roman goddess of agriculture and harvest.

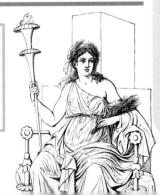

PICK IT

Nutritional Value

SERVING	1 cup
CALORIES	79
FAT	0 g
CARBS	15.8 g
FIBER	8 g
SUGAR	6 g
SODIUM	111 mg
PROTEIN	5 g

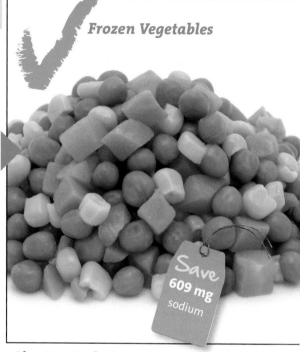

Frozen Vegetables

Save 609 mg sodium

❯ QUICK & EASY

Get the right amount:
Here are a few examples of servings of vegetables. Use them as a guide for eating five servings per day:

- One full cup of spinach
- Five florets of broccoli
- Ten baby carrots or one large carrot
- Half a baked sweet potato
- One plum tomato
- Six spears of asparagus
- Half a medium bell pepper
- Half a cup of squash

Give It a Try!

Frozen fruit (¾ cup)
60 calories, 0.7 g fat, 1 mg sodium

Grapes (1 cup)
62 calories, 0.3 g fat, 2 mg sodium

Steamfresh Selects mixed vegetables (1 cup)
90 calories, 0 fat, 30 mg sodium

Try This

To retain as many vitamins as possible, avoid thawing frozen vegetables before cooking. Simply start cooking them in their frozen state to preserve as much of their nutritional profile as possible.

❯❯ *FAST FACT*

By choosing vegetables of assorted colors you can significantly increase the number and kinds of anti-oxidants and phytochemicals you provide your body. Each color provides a different combination of these free-radical fighters.

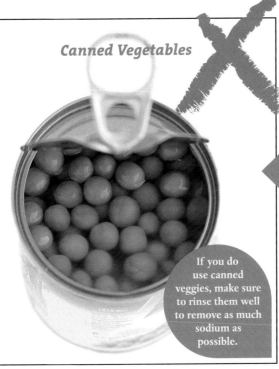

Canned Vegetables

KICK IT

Nutritional Value

SERVING	1 cup
CALORIES	80
FAT	0 g
CARBS	16 g
FIBER	4.9 g
SUGAR	6 g
SODIUM	720 mg
PROTEIN	4 g

If you do use canned veggies, make sure to rinse them well to remove as much sodium as possible.

HEALTH ALERT!

The linings of most vegetable cans are treated with assorted chemicals to help the cans retain integrity across a long shelf life. One of the substances, BPA, or bisphenol-A, has recently caused concern among scientists, who believe that this synthetic estrogen is a hormone disruptor responsible for assorted health problems, particularly for newborns and young children. It is highly recommended that pregnant women and young children avoid eating foods that have come into contact with BPA.

Ditch These Too!

Canned fruit cocktail (¾ cup)
103 calories, 0.2 g fat, 11 mg sodium

Canned grape juice (1 cup)
143 calories, 0 fat, 23 mg sodium

Chef Boyardee Beefaroni, canned (1 cup)
236 calories, 7 g fat, 959 mg sodium

 FAST FACT

MIX IT UP *No two vegetables contain similar nutrients and antioxidants. Nutritionists agree that eating a broad range of vegetables creates a synergy between the assorted nutrients that will go a long way toward promoting health and weight loss.*

PICK IT

Nutritional Value

SERVING	1 bar
CALORIES	190
FAT	9 g
CARBS	29 g
FIBER	5 g
SUGAR	21 g
SODIUM	0 mg
PROTEIN	4 g

> QUICK & EASY

Keep track of what you eat and drink every day. By writing down what you consume, you'll be able to tell if you need to eat more from any food groups or if you need to eat less of processed or high-fat foods.

Try This

Try to include a different fruit or vegetable in your meal each time you eat. Challenge yourself to try one new fruit or veggie each week. Check out new markets and grocery stores to broaden your horizons.

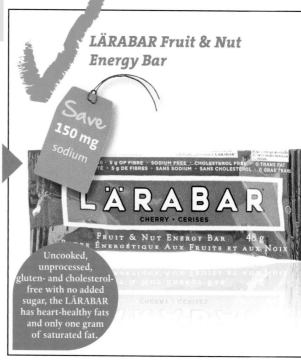

LÄRABAR Fruit & Nut Energy Bar

Save 150 mg sodium

LÄRABAR CHERRY • CERISES

FRUIT & NUT ENERGY BAR 48 g

Uncooked, unprocessed, gluten- and cholesterol-free with no added sugar, the LÄRABAR has heart-healthy fats and only one gram of saturated fat.

Give It a Try!

Newton 100% whole wheat fig cookies
130 calories, 2.5 g fat, 135 mg sodium

Ritz reduced-fat crackers (1 serving)
70 calories, 2 g fat, 150 mg sodium

Air-popped popcorn (1 cup)
31 calories, 0.4 g fat, 1 mg sodium

Say What?

SEVERAL RESEARCH STUDIES have found a link between cocoa and health benefits. Cocoa contains a large amount of antioxidants and it may also lower your risk of stroke and heart attacks by keeping blood pressure down and reducing the blood's ability to clot.

*PowerBar Triple Threat
Chocolate Caramel Fusion*

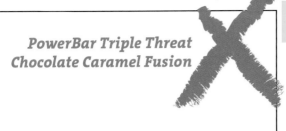

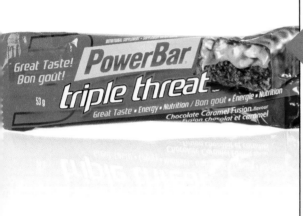

Nutritional Value	
SERVING	1 bar
CALORIES	230
FAT	8 g
CARBS	30 g
FIBER	4 g
SUGAR	15 g
SODIUM	150 mg
PROTEIN	10 g

ALL YOU!

Pinpoint the strengths and weaknesses in your current diet. Do you eat two and a half cups each of fruits and vegetables daily? Do you get enough calcium? Do you eat whole grain foods frequently? If so, you're on the right track! Keep it up. If not, add more of these foods to your daily diet.

Ditch These Too!

Oreo cookies (1 serving)
160 calories, 7 g fat, 190 mg sodium

Kraft Cheese Nips (1 serving)
150 calories, 6 g fat, 340 mg sodium

Trail mix (¼ cup)
150 calories, 10 g fat, 40 mg sodium

YES YOU CAN

Make exercise a habit by following these tips:
- Exercise at a certain time every day.
- Sign a contract that commits you to exercise regularly.
- Put "exercise dates" or "appointments" on your calendar.
- Check how you're progressing. Can you walk faster now than when you started? Or can you go for longer?
- Ask your doctor to write a prescription for an exercise program, which includes what kinds of exercises to do, how often to exercise and for how long.

Unsalted Pistachio Nuts

Nutritional Value	
SERVING	½ oz
CALORIES	79
FAT	6.3 g
CARBS	4 g
FIBER	1.5 g
SUGAR	1.1 g
SODIUM	0 mg
PROTEIN	2.9 g

Save
70 mg
sodium

Give It A Try!

✓ **Raw baby carrots (1 serving)**
30 calories, 0.1 g fat, 66 mg sodium

✓ **Sunflower seeds (¼ cup)**
186.5 calories, 16 g fat, 1 mg sodium

✓ **Raw unsalted almonds (½ oz)**
82 calories, 7 g fat, 0 sodium

BONUS!

Pistachio nuts are a great source of protein. Unsalted pistachios are high in potassium and low in sodium, which helps to keep blood pressure low, maintain water balance and strengthen muscles. Pistachio nuts are also a good source of vitamin E, which boosts the immune system and beats fatigue.

FATTER, NOT FITTER

Don't be fooled by the "Light" stamped on the box. Not only do the contents of the popcorn lack any nutritional value, just two cups of this snack has five grams of fat and 320 milligrams of sodium.

Per serving, pistachios have more antioxidants than green tea.

QUICK & EASY ▼

Have a dog? Walking is great exercise – do it daily and count it in. It's good for you and your pet.

 FAST FACT

Walking at a brisk pace (a 15-minute mile, or four mph) burns almost as many calories as jogging for the same distance, which may be too strenuous for some.

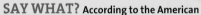

SAY WHAT? According to the American Association for Cancer Research Frontiers, a diet that incorporates a daily dose of pistachios may help reduce the risk of lung and other cancers. "Higher intake of gamma-tocopherol, which is a form of vitamin E, may reduce the risk of lung cancer," said Ladia M. Hernandez, M.S., R.D., L.D. "Pistachios are a good source of gamma-tocopherol ... so pistachios may help to decrease lung cancer risk," she says.

KICK IT ✗

Orville Redenbacher's Light Butter Popcorn

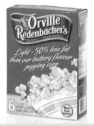

Nutritional Value

SERVING	2 cups
CALORIES	40
FAT	2 g
CARBS	8 g
FIBER	1 g
SUGAR	0 g
SODIUM	70 mg
PROTEIN	1 g

Ditch These Too! ↘

✗ **Lay's classic potato chips (1 oz)**
150 calories, 10 g fat, 180 g carbs

✗ **Tostitos tortilla chips (1 oz)**
140 calories, 7 g fat, 115 g carbs

✗ **Rold Gold pretzel sticks (1 oz)**
100 calories, 0 fat, 580 g carbs

PICK IT

Nutritional Value

SERVING	1.8 oz
CALORIES	60
FAT	0 g
CARBS	19 g
FIBER	0 g
SUGAR	2 g
SODIUM	240 mg
PROTEIN	3 g

A BETTER CHOICE

Trying to get active and exercise regularly? Go for a walk. Walking is considered one of the best exercise choices because it's easy, safe and inexpensive. Brisk walking can burn as much fat as jogging, but is less likely to cause injuries. Walking is both an aerobic and a weight-bearing exercise, so it's great for your heart and builds stronger bones.

Angelfood Cake

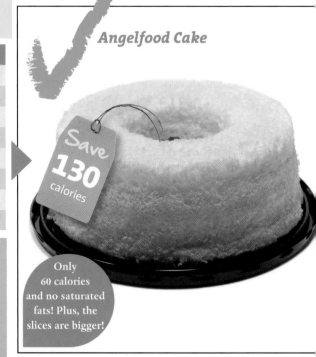

Save **130** calories

Only 60 calories and no saturated fats! Plus, the slices are bigger!

Give It a Try!

Jell-o gelatin desserts – strawberry (1 serving)
10 calories, 0 fat, 10 mg sodium

Fat-free Cool Whip (1 serving)
15 calories, 0 fat, 5 mg sodium

Klondike Slim-A-Bear premium fudge bar (1 serving)
100 calories, 3 g fat, 90 mg sodium

YES YOU CAN Don't drink empty calories. Drink no- or low-calorie beverages, such as water or un-sweetened tea. Avoid fruit drinks, regular soft drinks, sports drinks, energy drinks, sweetened or flavored milk, and sweetened iced tea. They add lots of sugar and calories to your diet with no nutritional value.

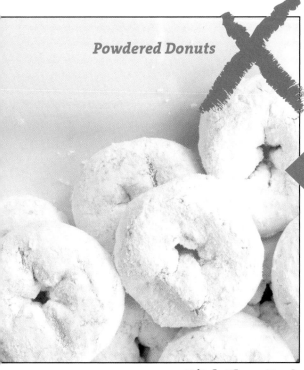

Powdered Donuts

KICK IT

Nutritional Value	
SERVING	1 donut (1.7 oz)
CALORIES	190
FAT	9 g
CARBS	25 g
FIBER	0 g
SUGAR	13 g
SODIUM	230 mg
PROTEIN	2 g

Try This

Finding it hard to lose those last five pounds? Try watching the amount of hidden fat and calories you consume. Scan the nutrition labels on foods before you buy them. Eliminate extra fat, such as butter or margarine on bread, sour cream on baked potatoes and salad dressings, by buying low-fat or nonfat versions or by skipping them altogether.

Ditch These Too!

Apple pie
411 calories, 19.4 g fat, 327 mg sodium

Vanilla ice cream (½ cup)
240 calories, 16 g fat, 60 mg sodium

Hershey's chocolate bar
210 calories, 13 g fat, 35 mg sodium

TIP Exercise for your overall health, not just to lose weight. Hitting the gym regularly reduces your risk of heart disease, high blood pressure, osteoporosis, diabetes and obesity. It also keeps you younger by reducing some of the effects of aging, and contributes to your mental health by boosting your energy and helping to treat depression.

65

Studies have suggested that by engaging in brisk walks for three or more hours a week, you can reduce your risk for coronary heart disease by 65 percent.

PICK IT

Nutritional Value	
SERVING	1 pop
CALORIES	100
FAT	2 g
CARBS	17 g
FIBER	1 g
SUGAR	14 g
SODIUM	75 mg
PROTEIN	2 g

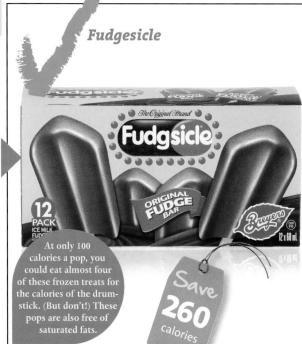

Fudgesicle

At only 100 calories a pop, you could eat almost four of these frozen treats for the calories of the drumstick. (But don't!) These pops are also free of saturated fats.

Save **260** calories

▶ QUICK & EASY

Make sure you fit in vitamin B12! Vitamin B12 is an important vitamin that you usually get in your daily diet. It is found mainly in fish, shellfish, meat and dairy products. Vitamin B12 helps make red blood cells and DNA, and maintains your nervous system. Most people with low vitamin B12 levels either do not consume meat and dairy products, or have trouble absorbing vitamin B12.

Give It a Try!

Fat-free chocolate fudge brownie ice cream (½ cup)
110 calories, 0 fat, 75 mg sodium

Vanilla frozen yogurt (½ cup)
120 calories, 4 g fat, 60 mg sodium

Skinny Cow vanilla and chocolate ice cream sandwich
140 calories, 1.5 g fat, 95 mg sodium

YES YOU CAN
Be a busy person who exercises! If you "don't have time" for a workout, then fit in mini-workouts, five to ten minutes each, several times throughout your day. Take the stairs, park your car further away from the office and count in household chores such as mowing the lawn, vacuuming or a short brisk walk around the block at lunch.

Nestlé Vanilla Fudge Drumstick

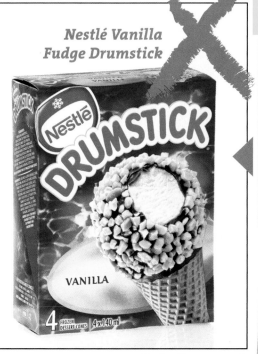

KICK IT

Nutritional Value	
SERVING	1 cone
CALORIES	360
FAT	21 g
CARBS	38 g
FIBER	0.5 g
SUGAR	23 g
SODIUM	110 mg
PROTEIN	5 g

Try This

Up your dietary fiber for better health! Fiber may help reduce your cholesterol and lower your risk of coronary heart disease, type 2 diabetes and certain types of cancer. What's more, it helps you to feel fuller longer. To increase the amount of fiber in your diet, eat vegetables such as beans, artichokes, sweet potatoes, peas, berries, prunes, figs and dates. Opt for whole grain breads and cereals instead of white bread. Eat brown rice instead of white rice. Bran muffins, oatmeal and bran cereals are also good sources of fiber.

Ditch These Too!

 Breyer's mint chocolate ice cream (½ cup)
150 calories, 8 g fat, 40 mg sodium

 Brownie
290 calories, 13 g fat, 150 mg sodium

 Cheesecake (1 piece)
257 calories, 18 g fat, 166 mg sodium

25 percentage of American adults — and an even greater percentage of women — are sedentary. After age 44, upwards of 30 percent of American women are sedentary.

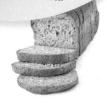

PICK IT

Nutritional Value

SERVING	1 bar
CALORIES	120
FAT	2 g
CARBS	24 g
FIBER	4 g
SUGAR	8 g
SODIUM	75 mg
PROTEIN	5 g

Kashi Chewy Granola Bars in Cherry Dark Chocolate

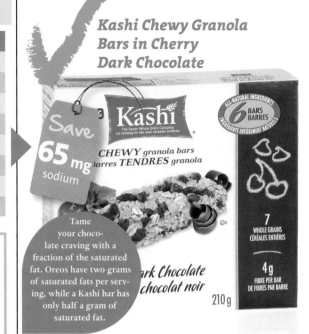

Save **65 mg** sodium

Tame your chocolate craving with a fraction of the saturated fat. Oreos have two grams of saturated fats per serving, while a Kashi bar has only half a gram of saturated fat.

>> FAST FACT

Be careful about the amount of sugar you consume. The American Heart Association advises that women consume no more than six teaspoons of added sugar a day (about 100 calories), about the same amount of sugar in a half cup serving of ice cream and less than the amount in one 12-ounce can of regular soda.

Give It a Try!

Almonds (1 oz)
164 calories, 14.3 g fat, 0 sodium

Slim-Fast peanut butter crunch bar
120 calories, 4.5 g fat, 80 mg sodium

Freshdirect fruit and yogurt snack pack
110 calories, 2 g fat, 75 mg sodium

YES YOU CAN Get toned without pulling a muscle. Strength training helps to prevent age-related bone and muscle-mass losses. Target areas where you want to build muscle tone, but don't neglect the other muscle groups. The phrase "no pain, no gain" is more often untrue. Start strength training slowly and build up to heavier weights and repetitions, especially if you are out of shape.

KICK IT

Oreo Cookies

Mr. Christie, you make good cookies!
M. Christie, vous faites de bons biscuits !

OREO

Chocolate Sandwich Cookies · Biscuits - sandwichs au chocolat

COOKIES ENLARGED TO SHOW TEXTURE
BISCUITS AGRANDIS POUR EN MONTRER LA TEXTURE

350 g

Nutritional Value	
SERVING	2 cookies
CALORIES	140
FAT	6.1 g
CARBS	21.9 g
FIBER	0.9 g
SUGAR	12.3 g
SODIUM	140 mg
PROTEIN	0.9 g

> QUICK & EASY

Limit your added sugar intake:

- Reduce your consumption of candy, sweets and baked goods.

- Opt instead for fruits, vegetables, lean proteins and whole grains for meals and snacks.

- Skip sugary drinks and choose water instead.

- Look for recipes for baked goods with low amounts of sugar.

Ditch These Too!

Nature Valley bar – oats n' honey
180 calories, 6 g fat, 160 mg sodium

Quaker Chewy bar – chocolate
140 calories, 5 g fat, 80 mg sodium

Larabar bar – cashew cookie
210 calories, 12 g fat, 0 sodium

Say What?

CHOCOLATE IS GOOD FOR YOU! Well, in moderation, that is. Research has shown that chocolate is a great source of antioxidants. Why are antioxidants important? These nutrients are believed to combat oxidative stress, which is associated with some neurodegenerative and cardiovascular diseases. Some studies also suggest that antioxidants help the body fight cancer.

PICK IT

Nutritional Value

SERVING	1.5 oz
CALORIES	190
FAT	10.4 g
CARBS	21.6 g
FIBER	1.7 g
SUGAR	17.3 g
SODIUM	9 mg
PROTEIN	3.5 g

❯ QUICK & EASY

Benefit from your chocolate fix by following these tips:

- Stay away from milk chocolate in order to benefit from chocolate nutrition – go for dark chocolate instead. Studies have shown that milk chocolate counteracts the effect of the antioxidants it contains.
- Drink water instead of milk after eating chocolate. Researchers suggest forgoing that glass of milk with chocolate, because milk interferes with how antioxidants in chocolate are absorbed.

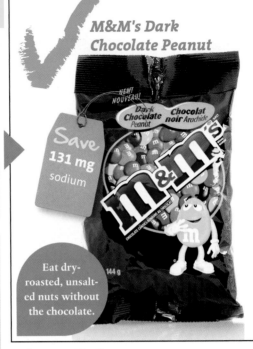

M&M's Dark Chocolate Peanut

Save **131 mg** sodium

Eat dry-roasted, unsalted nuts without the chocolate.

Give It a Try!

Slim-Fast creamy milk chocolate shake (1 can)
220 calories, 3 g fat, 220 mg sodium

Yoplait Whips! yogurt snack – chocolate
160 calories, 4 g fat, 105 mg sodium

Jell-o fat-free pudding – chocolate
100 calories, 0 fat, 180 mg sodium

YES YOU CAN

Work out without getting injured. **Balance exercises can help prevent falls and injuries.** Try fitting in exercises such as walking heel to toe, standing on one foot, or standing up and sitting down without using your hands. Also, don't neglect stretching: it helps you maintain your flexibility. Fit in 10 minutes of stretching twice a week to improve your flexibility and help prevent injuries.

Snickers Chocolate Bar

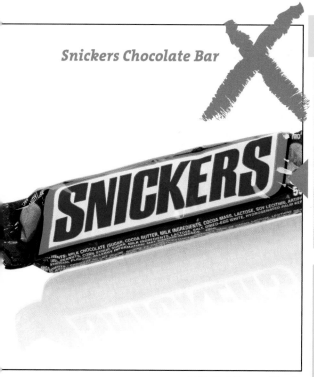

Nutritional Value	
SERVING	1 bar
CALORIES	280
FAT	14 g
CARBS	35 g
FIBER	1 g
SUGAR	30 g
SODIUM	140 mg
PROTEIN	4 g

❯ QUICK & EASY

Avoid trans fat.
It really is as bad for you as experts say. Ideally, you should get zero grams of trans fat per day. The American Heart Association recommends that no more than one percent of daily total calories should come from trans fat. So if you consume about 2,000 calories each day, you should eat less than two grams of trans fat per day. Try to reduce the amount of margarine, shortening, crackers, cookies and chips you eat. Reach for those veggies instead!

Ditch These Too!

Cadbury bar – fruit and nut
200 calories, 10 g fat, 30 mg sodium

Hershey's chocolate candies – special dark truffle (4 pieces)
220 calories, 13 g fat, 40 mg sodium

Dove Miniatures – milk chocolate
220 calories, 13 g fat, 25 mg sodium

A BETTER CHOICE

A powerhouse snack, edamame has more fiber than chips and can easily be portioned out into snack bags to take on the go. It also has healthy omega-3 fats! For a sweet treat, try dark-chocolate-covered edamame.

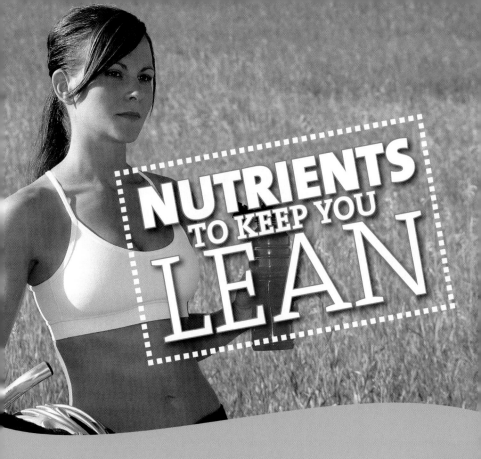

NUTRIENTS TO KEEP YOU LEAN

Nutrient	RDA/AI	Food Saver
Calcium	1,000 mg	1 cup tofu = 868 mg
Potassium	2,000 mg	1 cup sundried tomatoes = 1,851 mg
Fiber	25 g	1 endive = 16 g
Magnesium	320 mg	1 cup Swiss chard = 150 mg
Vitamin C	75 mg	1 cup broccoli = 81 mg
Vitamin E	15 mg	1 oz almonds = 7 mg

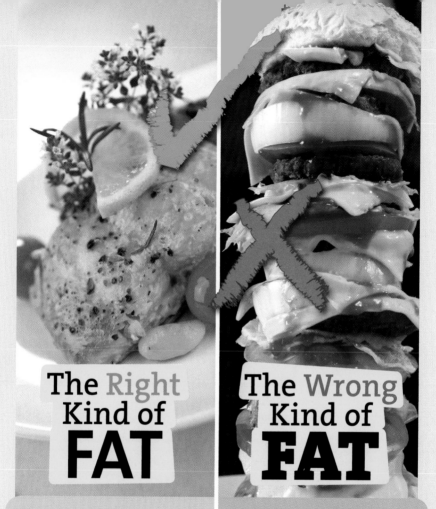

The Right Kind of FAT

If your fear of fat has you scouring nutrition labels for the best fat-free options, remember this: you need omega-3 fatty acids. Because of their anti-inflammatory properties, these healthy fats have proven heart health benefits and have also been attributed to reduced arthritis, age-related memory loss, incidences of diabetes and feelings of depression.

The Wrong Kind of FAT

Trans fats aren't your only enemy – so too are saturated fats, the ones that can raise your cholesterol. According to recent research, it just takes one super-saturated meal to affect the body's ability to protect its arteries against plaque. According to the American Heart Association, your daily intake shouldn't exceed seven percent of total calories.

PICK IT

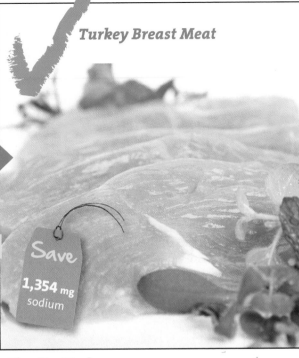

Turkey Breast Meat

Nutritional Value

SERVING	4 oz
CALORIES	153
FAT	0.8 g
CARBS	0 g
FIBER	0 g
SUGAR	0 g
SODIUM	59 mg
PROTEIN	34 g

Save 1,354 mg sodium

BONUS!

Turkey is a

great source of protein. A four-ounce serving provides about 65 percent of the daily value for protein.

MAKE IT BETTER

Get the tryptophan without the extra calories! Cut the serving in half and have half a turkey sandwich before bedtime.

1,440

The number of minutes in every day. Set aside 30 of them for physical activity!

Give It a Try!

Shrimp (4 large)
22 calories, 0.2 g fat, 49 mg sodium

Light tuna, canned in water (1 can)
80 calories, 1 g fat, 50 mg sodium

Extra lean ham, sliced
69 calories, 1.8 g fat, 697 mg sodium

Say What?

TURKEY IS A VERY GOOD SOURCE of selenium, a mineral that is of major importance to your overall health. Accumulated evidence from several research studies have suggested an inverse correlation between selenium intake and cancer incidence.

Roast Chicken Deli Meat

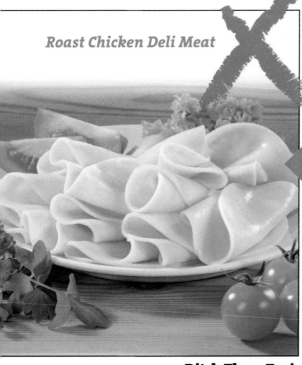

KICK IT

Nutritional Value	
SERVING	4 oz
CALORIES	122
FAT	3.5 g
CARBS	1.7 g
FIBER	0 g
SUGAR	1.7 g
SODIUM	1,413 mg
PROTEIN	19.2 g

A BETTER CHOICE

Turn off the television and make family time physically active. Plan a weekend bike ride, fit in a family baseball game or take an evening walk around the block.

Ditch These Too!

Italian sausage, cooked (1 link)
230 calories, 18.3 g fat, 809 mg sodium

Oscar Meyer center cut bacon (1 serving)
50 calories, 4 g fat, 270 mg sodium

Beef hot dog (1 serving)
149 calories, 13.3 g fat, 513 mg sodium

Try This

Motivate yourself to exercise regularly by finding the right exercise for you. If it's fun, you are more likely to commit to it. You may want to hike with a friend, join a class or plan a group bike ride.

MAKE IT **BETTER**

Your diet can help your immune system. Try adding foods that contain probiotics – live micro-organisms. Research shows that these microscopic organisms may help treat a myriad of digestive problems.

PICK IT

Nutritional Value	
SERVING	1 cup
CALORIES	120
FAT	2 g
CARBS	12 g
FIBER	3 g
SUGAR	8 g
SODIUM	125 mg
PROTEIN	14 g

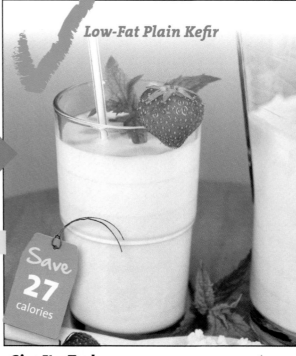

Low-Fat Plain Kefir

Save **27** calories

BONUS!

Kefir contains lactic acid bacteria. Research has shown that probiotic bacteria, like the kinds found in kefir, are good for people with common gastrointestinal upsets such as lactose intolerance, irritable bowel syndrome, constipation and diarrhea.

 FAST FACT

The word kefir (pronounced keh-FEER) is said to have its origins in the Turkish word for "well-being." It has long been used in Russia for treating ailments ranging from stomach ulcers to pneumonia. Kefir is made by combining milk with beneficial bacteria.

Give It a Try!

Yoplait light yogurt (1 pot)
100 calories, 0 fat, 85 mg sodium

Mozzarella partly skimmed milk cheese (1 oz)
72 calories, 4.5 g fat, 175 mg sodium

Light vanilla soymilk (1 cup)
80 calories, 2 g fat, 95 mg sodium

Say What?

KEFIR IS LOW IN CALORIES, and high in protein and calcium. One serving of plain, nonfat kefir has only 87 calories while providing 10.5 grams of protein and 20 percent of the daily value for calcium. It's also a good source of magnesium, riboflavin, folate and vitamin B-12.

Whole Milk

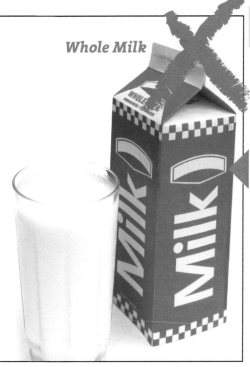

Nutritional Value	
SERVING	1 cup
CALORIES	147
FAT	8.1 g
CARBS	12.9 g
FIBER	0 g
SUGAR	12.9 g
SODIUM	98 mg
PROTEIN	7.9 g

❯ QUICK & EASY

Enjoy kefir throughout the day:

BREAKFAST
Blend up a powerful probiotic smoothie with half a banana, a half-cup of blueberries and a half-cup of low-fat kefir.

LUNCH
Stir a quarter cup of plain kefir into a creamy bowl of butternut squash soup. Enjoy with a sandwich made with toasted whole grain bread.

DINNER
Instead of sour cream, spoon thickened kefir onto a baked potato for a probiotic boost. Top with chives and serve alongside a grilled steak and side salad.

Ditch These Too!

Salted butter (1 Tbsp)
102 calories, 11.5 g fat, 82 mg sodium

Whole yogurt (1 cup)
149 calories, 8.1 g fat, 10 mg sodium

Feta cheese (1 wedge)
100 calories, 8.1 g fat, 424 mg sodium

ALL YOU!

Get stronger muscles for stronger bones. Exercise in any form is great for you and can help reduce the risk of disease. But when it comes to strengthening your bones, milder forms of activity may not be enough. Researchers concluded that overall aerobic fitness and mild physical activity did not have a significant effect on bone density. Greater muscle strength, however, was associated with stronger bones – so pick up those weights!

PICK IT

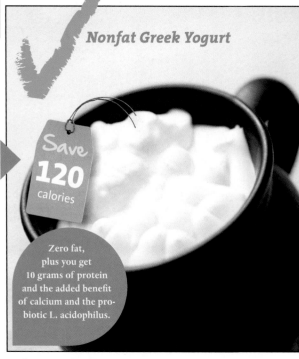

Nonfat Greek Yogurt

Save
120
calories

Zero fat, plus you get 10 grams of protein and the added benefit of calcium and the probiotic L. acidophilus.

Nutritional Value	
SERVING	½ cup
CALORIES	60
FAT	0 g
CARBS	3.5 g
FIBER	0 g
SUGAR	3 g
SODIUM	35 mg
PROTEIN	11 g

 FAST FACT

Greek yogurt has a low-sugar and a high-protein content, which, among other benefits, makes you feel full for longer.

> **QUICK & EASY**

SAVORY: Mix Greek yogurt with one or two tablespoons of Knorr Soup Mix and have it as an afternoon snack with sliced cucumber and peppers.

SWEET: Add a half cup of Kashi GoLean cereal to Greek yogurt, along with a sprinkle of cinnamon and one teaspoon of ground flaxseed, for a healthier version of a yogurt parfait.

Give It a Try!
Dannon Light n' Fit nonfat vanilla yogurt
80 calories, 0 fat, 75 mg sodium

Light swiss cheese (1 serving)
35 calories, 2 g fat, 260 mg sodium

Fat-free cream cheese (1 oz)
27 calories, 0.4 g fat, 155 mg sodium

BONUS!

Greek yogurt has a smooth, rich and thick consistency that is delicious and nutritious. Part of what makes Greek yogurt different from regular yogurt is that it is strained to remove the whey, giving it a dense texture.

Full-Fat Cottage Cheese

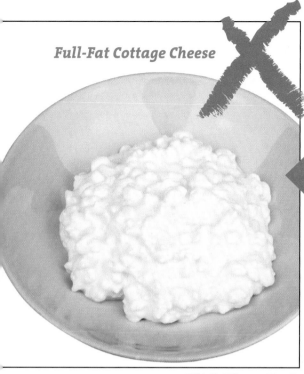

KICK IT

Ditch These Too!

Cheddar cheese (slice)
113 calories, 9.3 g fat, 174 mg sodium

Cream cheese (1 oz)
99 calories, 9.9 g fat, 84 mg sodium

Parmesan shredded cheese (1 Tbsp)
21 calories, 1.4 g fat, 85 mg sodium

Get more calcium by making simple changes. Choose low-fat yogurt or low-fat cheese with fruit as a snack. You can also try calcium-rich beverages such as calcium-fortified orange juice and soymilk, and goat's milk. Tofu and canned fish with bones are also high in calcium. By including these foods into your diet, you can have a calcium-rich diet without needing supplements.

EXCUSE BUSTED

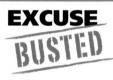

Bored by your exercise routine?

- **Bring a friend** to work out with. If your buddy is on the next bike or treadmill, your workout will be less boring.

- **Watch TV or listen to music** while you walk or pedal indoors. Another great idea: check out audio books from your local library.

- **Get outside.** A change in scenery can stimulate you to work out harder.

PICK IT

Nutritional Value

SERVING	1 cup
CALORIES	2
FAT	0 g
CARBS	0.5 g
FIBER	0 g
SUGAR	0.1 g
SODIUM	0 mg
PROTEIN	0 g

TIP Hydrate, hydrate, hydrate. After sweating it out during an intense workout, you may easily need an additional quart of water. You will also need additional water whenever you have obvious water loss, as would occur with even fairly mild diarrhea. Consume water in a somewhat regular pattern and keep your water intake adequate throughout the day.

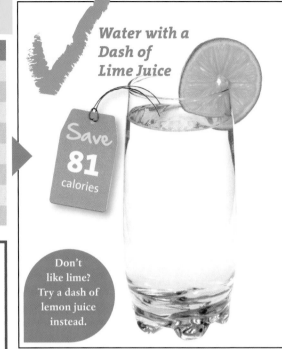

Water with a Dash of Lime Juice

Save **81** calories

Don't like lime? Try a dash of lemon juice instead.

Give It a Try!

V8 low-sodium vegetable juice (8 oz)
50 calories, 0 fat, 140 mg sodium

Natural green tea (1 tea bag)
0 calories, 0 fat, 0 sodium

Perrier water
0 calories, 0 fat, 0 sodium

YES YOU CAN Drink up for a healthier heart. One research study determined that adults drinking five or more glasses of water each day were about 50 percent less likely to die from a heart attack than those who did not. The researchers involved in this study ranked increased water intake very close in importance to stopping smoking in terms of heart health.

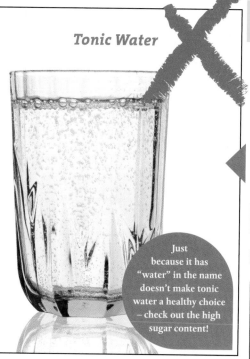

Tonic Water

Nutritional Value	
SERVING	1 cup
CALORIES	83
FAT	0 g
CARBS	21.5 g
FIBER	0 g
SUGAR	21.5 g
SODIUM	29 mg
PROTEIN	0 g

Just because it has "water" in the name doesn't make tonic water a healthy choice – check out the high sugar content!

TIP Take in potassium to help your body maintain healthy blood pressure. The USDA recommends that the average American consume 4,044 milligrams of potassium each day. You can up your potassium intake by eating the following foods: sweet potatoes, white beans, soybeans, lima beans and kidney beans, nonfat yogurt, skim milk; or fruit such as bananas, peaches, cantaloupe; or fish such as halibut, yellowfin tuna and cod.

Ditch These Too!
Coca-Cola Classic
97 calories, 0 fat, 31 mg sodium

Sugar-free Red Bull
11 calories, 0 fat, 204 mg sodium

Gatorade energy drink
50 calories, 0 fat, 200 mg sodium

Say What?

WE CAN GO FAR LONGER without food than without water, and all of our nutrient requirements are affected by the amount of water we drink. The reason is simple: our bodies are about 60 percent water by weight and most nutrients travel through our body in water. There isn't a bodily function that does not depend on water, so drink up!

Chamomile Tea

Save
108
calories

Nutritional Value	
SERVING	1 cup
CALORIES	0
FAT	0 g
CARBS	0 g
FIBER	0 g
SUGAR	0 g
SODIUM	0 mg
PROTEIN	0 g

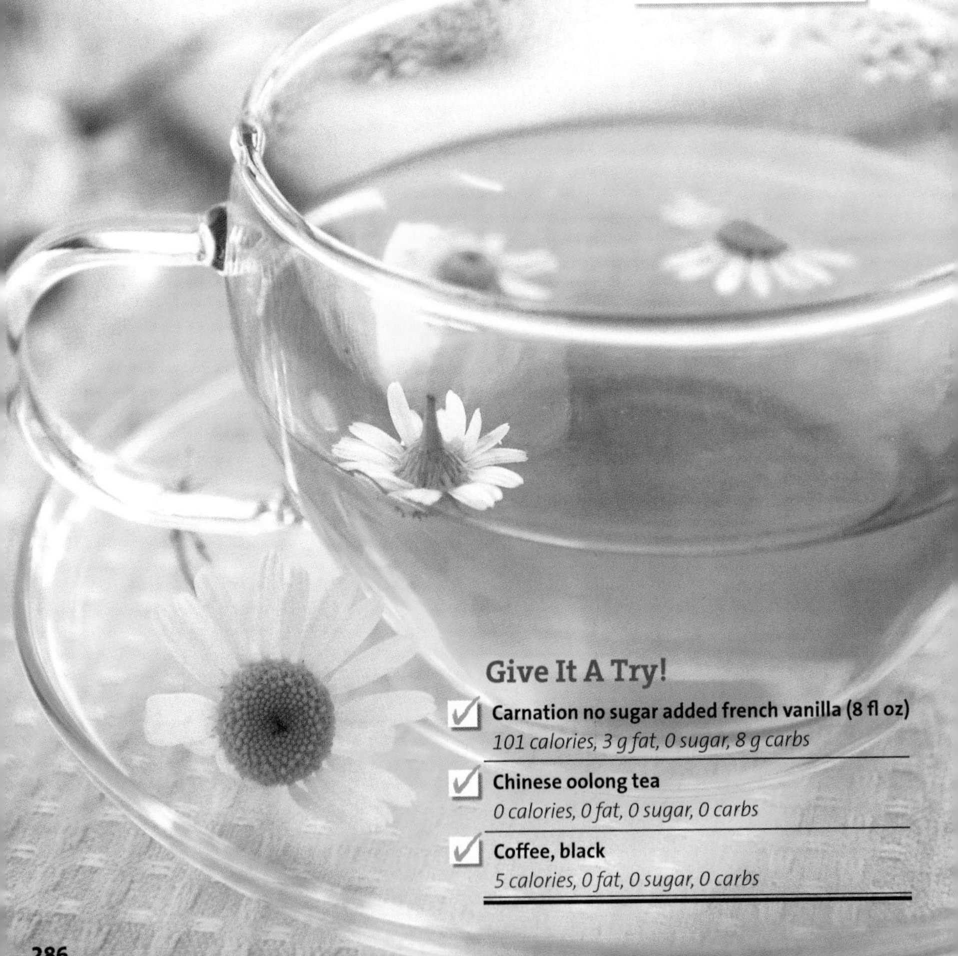

Give It A Try!

☑ **Carnation no sugar added french vanilla (8 fl oz)**
101 calories, 3 g fat, 0 sugar, 8 g carbs

☑ **Chinese oolong tea**
0 calories, 0 fat, 0 sugar, 0 carbs

☑ **Coffee, black**
5 calories, 0 fat, 0 sugar, 0 carbs

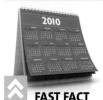

A Better Choice

Skip the burst of sugar and caffeine that will leave you crashing and jittery later. Herbal teas are caffeine free and offer a calming effect.

2010

FAST FACT

It takes about 12 weeks after beginning a regular workout program to notice measurable changes in your body and your overall health. However, before 12 weeks, you will notice that your strength and endurance have increased.

BONUS!

Research has found that chamomile tea can protect the body from both colds and menstrual cramps. According to a report in the *Journal of Agricultural and Food Chemistry*, chamomile functions as an anti-inflammatory, sedative and ulcer-fighter. Studies also suggest that chamomile may act as an antimicrobial and an antioxidant.

In Europe, chamomile is used to combat a host of conditions including sleep disorders, anxiety, skin infections/inflammation (including eczema), colic, teething pains and diaper rash. Most Americans sip chamomile tea for another reason – its reputed mild sedating effects.

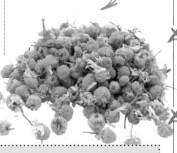

SAY WHAT? Chamomile may help to combat stress and depression by relaxing the brain. It can also be used to help insomnia by relaxing muscles and acting as a mild sedative. The tea also contains essential oils that help to heal skin irritations such as bites, stings and burns, and may even alleviate acne.

KICK IT

Energy Drinks

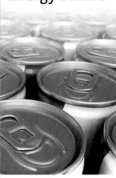

Nutritional Value

SERVING	8 fl oz
CALORIES	108
FAT	0 g
CARBS	27 g
FIBER	0 g
SUGAR	26.3 g
SODIUM	196 mg
PROTEIN	0.3 g

Ditch These Too!

Her energy drink (8 fl oz)
130 calories, 0 fat, 31 g sugar, 32 g carbs

SoBe Energy (8 fl oz)
120 calories, 0 fat, 31 g sugar, 32 g carbs

Full Throttle (8 fl oz)
110 calories, 0 fat, 29 g sugar, 29 g carbs

PICK IT

Nutritional Value

SERVING	1 cup
CALORIES	110
FAT	0 g
CARBS	26 g
FIBER	0 g
SUGAR	22 g
SODIUM	0 mg
PROTEIN	0 g

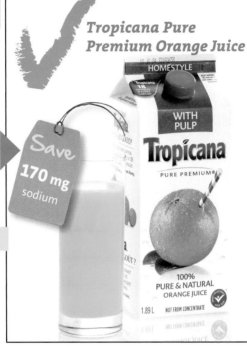

Tropicana Pure Premium Orange Juice

Save **170 mg** sodium

BONUS!

Drink it up!

Drinking that glass of orange juice in the morning may be better for you than taking vitamin C alone. One Italian research study found that consuming vitamin C supplements does not provide the same protective benefits as drinking a glass of orange juice.

TIP Fresh is best! For the best DNA protection, skip the vitamin C-fortified bottled drinks and enjoy a glass of real freshly squeezed orange juice – or simply eat an orange!

Give It a Try!

Tropicana calcium-enriched orange juice (1 cup)
108 calories, 0 fat, 0 sodium

Grapefruit juice (1 cup)
96 calories, 0.2 g fat, 2 mg sodium

Low-sodium tomato juice (1 cup)
50 calories, 0 fat, 140 mg sodium

YES YOU CAN

KEEP FIT WITHOUT BREAKING THE BANK.

Choose free activities. Take your kids to the park for a walk or bike ride.

Check out your local recreation or community center. Centers such as the YMCA may cost less than other gyms.

Choose physical activities that do not require special gear. Walking, jogging and running require only a pair of sturdy shoes.

KICK IT

SunnyD Original

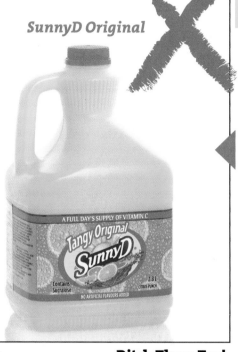

Nutritional Value	
SERVING	1 cup
CALORIES	130
FAT	0 g
CARBS	32 g
FIBER	0 g
SUGAR	30 g
SODIUM	170 mg
PROTEIN	0 g

A BETTER CHOICE

Orange juice has far more nutrients than orange drinks. SunnyD is not much more than high fructose corn syrup and water. Picking 100 percent fruit juices means you get more vitamins and the sugars are natural. Always pick orange juice over orange drink.

Ditch These Too!

Ginger ale (1 can)
124 calories, 0 fat, 26 mg sodium

Lipton iced tea (8 oz)
70 calories, 0 fat, 5 mg sodium

Tropicana cranberry cocktail
140 calories, 0 fat, 25 mg sodium

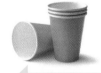

BONUS!

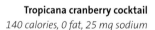

Research has shown that consumption

of vegetables and fruits high in vitamin C is associated with a reduced risk of death from such causes as heart disease, stroke and cancer. Orange juice can also decrease your risk of developing rheumatoid arthritis and kidney stones. A study published in the *British Journal of Nutrition* found that when women drank one-half to one liter of orange, grapefruit or apple juice daily, their urinary pH value and citric acid excretion increased, lowering their risk of forming kidney stones.

PICK IT

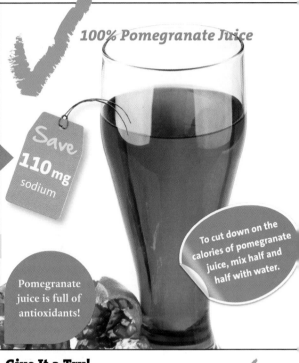

100% Pomegranate Juice

Nutritional Value	
SERVING	8 oz
CALORIES	160
FAT	0 g
CARBS	40 g
FIBER	0 g
SUGAR	34 g
SODIUM	10 mg
PROTEIN	0 g

Save **110 mg** sodium

To cut down on the calories of pomegranate juice, mix half and half with water.

Pomegranate juice is full of antioxidants!

BONUS!

Pomegranate fruits contain polyphenols, tannins and anthocyanins, all of which are beneficial antioxidants. The antioxidant levels in pomegranates are higher than most other fruit juices, red wine or green tea.

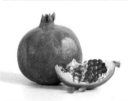

Give It a Try!

Pineapple juice (1 cup)
130 calories, 0 fat, 10 mg sodium

Grape juice (1 cup)
170 calories, 0 fat, 20 mg sodium

Prune juice (1 can)
122 calories, 0 fat, 20 mg sodium ✓

» FAST FACT

You're not alone in your quest to shed the pounds! At any given time, 33 percent to 40 percent of all American women are trying to lose weight.

Say What?

RESEARCH SUGGESTS that drinking concentrated pomegranate juice may reduce cholesterol. A clinical study in *Clinical Nutrition* suggested that drinking one glass of pomegranate juice a day for one year reduced blood pressure and slowed down "bad" cholesterol.

Fruit Punch Drink

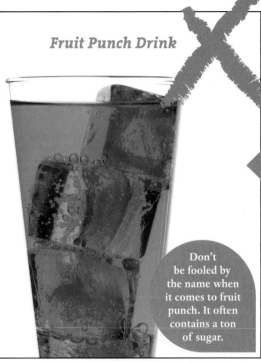

KICK IT

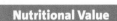

Nutritional Value	
SERVING	1 cup
CALORIES	120
FAT	0 g
CARBS	30 g
FIBER	0 g
SUGAR	29 g
SODIUM	120 mg
PROTEIN	0 g

Don't be fooled by the name when it comes to fruit punch. It often contains a ton of sugar.

Try This

Look for foods displaying the American Heart Association's heart-check mark to quickly pinpoint heart-healthy foods in the supermarket. The heart-check mark on food packaging indicates that the food has been certified to meet the American Heart Association's criteria for saturated fat and cholesterol for healthy people over age two.

Ditch These Too!

Kool-Aid Bursts – tropical punch (1 serving)
100 calories, 0 fat, 35 mg sodium

Starbucks caffe latte (with whole milk)
204 calories, 10.5 g fat, 156 mg sodium

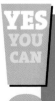

Fresca (1 can)
2 calories, 0 fat, 24 mg sodium

YES YOU CAN

Exercise and fit in quality time with your family. Do something physically active with your kids – they need physical activity too. No matter what age your kids are, find an activity you can do together. Dance to music, take a walk, run around the park, go skiing or play a pick-up game of basketball or soccer.

PICK IT

Nutritional Value	
SERVING	1 cup
CALORIES	91
FAT	0.7 g
CARBS	12.3 g
FIBER	0 g
SUGAR	12.3 g
SODIUM	130 mg
PROTEIN	8.7 g

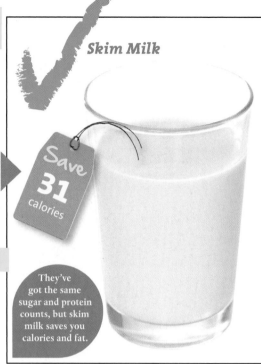

Skim Milk

Save **31** calories

They've got the same sugar and protein counts, but skim milk saves you calories and fat.

BONUS!

Fat-free milk

is high in protein and calcium, and contains a bevy of B vitamins. All this for only 86 calories in an eight-ounce glass! In fact, merely switching from whole milk to fat-free milk can be one of the more significant choices you can make in reducing saturated fat and calories in your diet.

Give It a Try!

Astro fat-free yogurt (1 serving)
60 calories, 0 fat, 75 mg sodium

Almond Breeze – unsweetened vanilla
40 calories, 3 g fat, 80 mg sodium

Yoplait Light yogurt – apricot mango
100 calories, 0 fat, 85 mg sodium

Say What?

RESEARCH HAS FOUND that a diet rich in fruits and vegetables plus three cups of milk or yogurt per day increased people's weight loss and helped them manage their weight better. A study indicated that calcium-rich dairy products helped people lose more weight from the abdominal region (stomach area) than those either taking calcium supplements or eating a low-calcium diet.

KICK IT

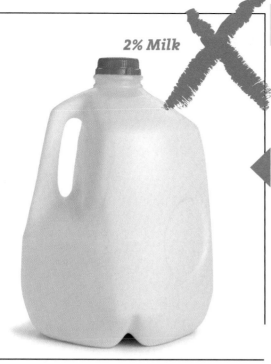

2% Milk

Nutritional Value

SERVING	1 cup
CALORIES	122
FAT	4.9 g
CARBS	12.5 g
FIBER	0 g
SUGAR	12.4 g
SODIUM	100 mg
PROTEIN	8.1 g

 FAST FACT

Dietary Guidelines recommend everyone aged nine years and older consume the equivalent of three cups of milk per day.

Ditch These Too!

Astro original yogurt (1 serving)
120 calories, 5 g fat, 55 mg sodium

Almond Breeze – chocolate
*120 calories, 2.5 g fat,
20 g sugar, 50 mg sodium*

Vanilla milkshake
717 calories, 22 g fat, 309 mg sodium

 YES YOU CAN

Be motivated to work out even if you're surrounded by inactive people. Remind yourself of the rewards you get from working out: better sleep, a happier mood, more energy and a stronger body.

Join a class or sports league where you'll be with other motivated, active people. Playing a game of basketball or joining a dance class is a great way of associating with people who regularly exercise and who will motivate you to get active too!

PICK IT

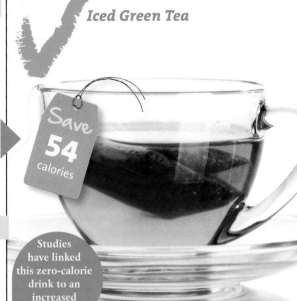

Iced Green Tea

Nutritional Value	
SERVING	1 cup
CALORIES	43
FAT	0 g
CARBS	10.3 g
FIBER	0 g
SUGAR	10.3 g
SODIUM	5 mg
PROTEIN	0 g

Save **54** calories

BONUS!

Green tea

drinkers appear to have a lower risk for developing a wide range of diseases, from simple bacterial or viral infections to chronic degenerative conditions including cardiovascular disease, cancer, stroke, periodontal disease and osteoporosis.

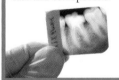

Studies have linked this zero-calorie drink to an increased metabolism!

Give It a Try!

Lipton green tea – mixed berry
0 calories, 0 fat, 70 mg sodium

Orange pekoe tea
35 calories, 0 fat, 0 sodium

Stash organic tea – white and raspberry
0 calories, 0 fat, 0 sodium

YES YOU CAN!

PREVENT THE HEAT OR THE COLD FROM GETTING YOU DOWN.
Keep active even in the most inclement weather by following the tips below:

- **Walk around the mall.** Join a local mall-walking group or club to walk indoors year-round.
- Sign up for a membership at a **fitness or community center.**
- **Exercise at home.** Work out to fitness videos or DVDs, or to your favourite MP3 playlists.

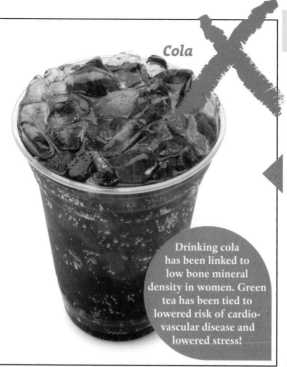

Cola

KICK IT

Nutritional Value	
SERVING	1 cup
CALORIES	97
FAT	0 g
CARBS	27 g
FIBER	0 g
SUGAR	27 g
SODIUM	33 mg
PROTEIN	0 g

Drinking cola has been linked to low bone mineral density in women. Green tea has been tied to lowered risk of cardiovascular disease and lowered stress!

Try This

If you simply cannot start your day without a cup of coffee, try enjoying a cup of green tea at your mid-morning break, with lunch or as an afternoon pick-me-up. You'll quickly discover green tea's irresistible combination of invigorating and calming qualities, plus its delicious flavor.

Ditch These Too!

Mountain Dew (8 oz)
108 calories, 0 fat, 49 mg sodium

X

Beer (1 can)
153 calories, 0 fat, 14 mg sodium

X

Fanta orange
110 calories, 0 fat, 35 mg sodium

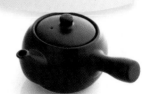

BONUS!

In August 2006, a European study published in the *European Journal of Clinical Nutrition* found that herbal tea is a healthier choice than almost any beverage. Tea not only rehydrates as well as water does, but provides a rich supply of polyphenols to protect against heart disease.

FOODS FOR MORE >> ENERGY!

10 Ways to Get More Energy from Your Food

Maximize your energy by knowing how to choose and prepare the right foods for you. Keep the following tips in mind:

1 Choose fresh from the garden whenever possible: foods in their natural state retain more nutrients than processed versions.

2 Include a variety of foods at every meal instead of the same combinations of cereal and fruit, for example. Vary the fruit (chopped apple instead of berries) and the cereal (oatmeal instead of bran cereal every day) and you will get more nutrients and minerals.

3 Pick dark, colorful vegetables over lighter varieties, as they contain more nutrients.

4 Choose whole fruits over fruit juice whenever possible for more fiber and nutritional value.

5 At the office, use powdered milk in your coffee in place of artificial creamers.

6 Hydrate your body throughout the day and during your workouts. If you eat lots of low-water snacks such as protein bars or dried fruit, dehydration might be sapping your energy.

7 Buy local, organic fruits and vegetables and you'll also avoid chemical pesticides, especially in apples, cherries, celery, imported grapes, nectarines, peaches, pears, strawberries and spinach, which are known to have higher pesticide residue.

8 Include small amounts of healthy fats in each meal to keep you feeling full longer: peanut butter, nut butters, olive oil and flaxseed make good choices.

9 Keep frozen fruits like bananas (peeled and cut into coins) on hand for a ready snack source or as an ingredient in smoothies.

10 Try dried fruits and trail mixes for good sources of potassium and carbohydrates.

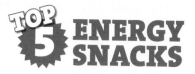

TOP 5 ENERGY SNACKS

Try these quick and tasty combos before or after your workout, when you're rushed at work, or while running errands on the weekend or evenings.

- Whole grain toast with almond butter
- Whole wheat pita with hummus
- Cottage cheese with pineapple
- Whole grain cereal with milk
- Low-fat cheese with fruit

BONUS IDEA: Chocolate milk

More Round-the-Clock Energy

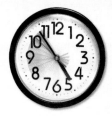

8:00 Breakfast

Energy-sustaining choices: milk and whole grain cereal, toast with peanut butter and fruit, egg whites and vegetables.

12:00 Lunch

Energy-sustaining choices: turkey on whole wheat bread, water-packed tuna and a vegetable salad, chicken and brown rice.

3:00 Mid-Afternoon

Energy-sustaining choices: tuna with steamed vegetables, turkey burger with a yam, pasta and salmon salad.

7:00 Dinner

Energy-sustaining choices: chicken and bulgur, salmon and vegetables, lean beef and brown rice.

Note:

Your meals may be further broken down into five or six smaller meals by eating half of any one meal before your workout and the other half after your workout.

PICK IT

Nutritional Value	
SERVING	20 chips
CALORIES	120
FAT	3 g
CARBS	21 g
FIBER	2 g
SUGAR	0 g
SODIUM	120 mg
PROTEIN	2 g

BONUS!

Baked and

kettle-cooked chips are available as healthier alternatives to deep-fried chips. Kettle-cooked chips are still fried in fats and oils, but contain more potato, which means more potato nutrients.

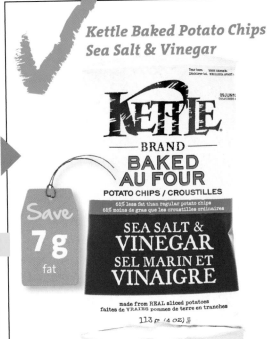

Kettle Baked Potato Chips Sea Salt & Vinegar

Give It a Try!

Skinny natural corn chips
120 calories, 2 g fat, 115 mg sodium

Quaker rice cakes – caramel corn
50 calories, 0 fat, 30 mg sodium

Special K bar – strawberry
90 calories, 1.5 g fat, 95 mg sodium

Say What?

MADE WITH WHOLE GRAINS. Many products make a whole grain claim even though they often consist mainly of refined flour with a minimal amount of whole grains. Read the nutrition label to be sure of what you're eating!

KICK IT

Lay's Potato Chips

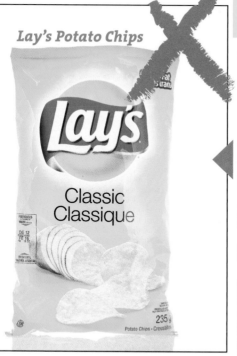

TIP When choosing high-calorie foods such as chips, take a portion and put it into a small bowl. Close the bag and put it back in to the cupboard before you start snacking.

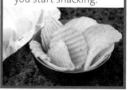

Ditch These Too!

Rold Gold pretzels (1 oz)
110 calories, 1 g fat, 580 mg sodium

Cheetos crunchy cheese snacks (1 oz)
160 calories, 10 g fat, 290 mg sodium

Chex Mix (1 oz)
120 calories, 4 g fat, 290 mg sodium

>> FAST FACT

Despite the proven benefits of physical activity, more than 60 percent of American adults do not get enough physical activity to provide health benefits, and more than 25 percent of adults are totally inactive in their leisure time.

YES YOU CAN
Exercise is great for your heart! A large-scale, six-year study involving 39,372 American women over age 44 shows that exercise reduces the risk of coronary heart disease. The study found that the more energy the women spent exercising, the lower their risk of developing this illness.

PICK IT

Nutritional Value

SERVING	1 oz
CALORIES	185
FAT	18.5 g
CARBS	3.9 g
FIBER	1.9 g
SUGAR	0.7 g
SODIUM	1 mg
PROTEIN	4.3 g

MAKE IT BETTER

Add walnuts to your diet to make your meals tastier and keep you feeling fuller for longer. Add walnuts to your morning cereal, add them to baked treats or toss them in a salad.

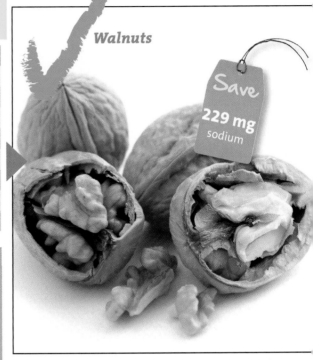

Walnuts

Save
229 mg
sodium

Give It a Try!

Cashew nuts (1 oz)
156 calories, 12.4 g fat, 3 mg sodium

Pumpkin and squash seeds (1 oz)
148 calories, 11.9 g fat, 5 mg sodium

Flaxseed (1 oz)
140 calories, 9 g fat, 0 sodium

TOP CHOICE! *Walnuts*

Walnuts not only taste great, they have a whole slew of health benefits, too! Rich in polyunsaturated fatty acids, walnuts may improve blood lipids and reduce other risk factors for cardiovascular disease. Eating walnuts regularly improves bone health and improves blood flow for those suffering from diabetes.

DID YOU KNOW?
Walnuts are the oldest tree food known to man (7,000 B.C.).

Roasted Salted Peanuts

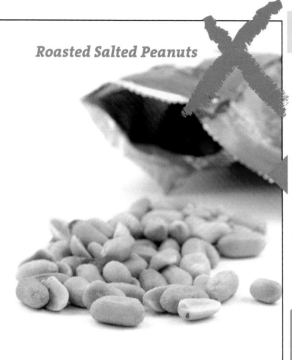

KICK IT

Nutritional Value	
SERVING	1 oz
CALORIES	166
FAT	14.1 g
CARBS	6.1 g
FIBER	2.3 g
SUGAR	1.2 g
SODIUM	230 mg
PROTEIN	6.7 g

ALL YOU!

Want great skin? You'd be better off eating that paste of crushed nuts, berries and yogurt, rather than slathering it on your face. Researchers found that those who follow a diet comprised mostly of fruits, vegetables, whole grains and unsaturated fats had noticeably smoother skin than those who consumed a fat- and sugar-laden diet. Antioxidants in these foods, including vitamins A, C and E, may help to protect the skin from environmental stress and damage.

Ditch These Too!

Pecans (1 oz)
196 calories, 20.4 g fat, 0 sodium

Salted macadamia nuts (1 oz)
203 calories, 21.5 g fat, 75 mg sodium

Dried Brazil nuts (1 oz)
186 calories, 18.8 g fat, 1 mg sodium

Say What?

YO-YO DIETING A study published in the *International Journal of Obesity* found that overweight participants who ate walnuts as part of a healthy diet did not gain weight. Participants who followed a Mediterranean-style diet including walnuts lost weight faster and were able to keep it off for longer than those following a typical low-fat diet.

Ben & Jerry's
Cherry Garcia Frozen Yogurt

Nutritional Value	
SERVING	½ cup
CALORIES	170
FAT	3 g
CARBS	32 g
FIBER	0.5 g
SUGAR	22 g
SODIUM	65 mg
PROTEIN	4 g

Save 100 calories

500 ml

BEN & JERRY'S

Don't Desert Dessert!
Ne désertez pas le dessert!

Cherry Garcia

Low Fat Frozen Yogurt
Yogourt glacé Faible en Gras

Cherry Frozen Yogourt with Cherries & Fudge Flakes
Yogourt glacé à la cerise truffé de cerises et de flocons de fudge

Give It A Try!

✓ **Jell-o pudding – dark chocolate tuxedo (1 serving)**
60 calories, 1.5 g fat, 180 mg sodium

✓ **Orange sherbet (½ cup)**
120 calories, 1 g fat, 35 mg sodium

✓ **No sugar added rice pudding (½ cup)**
70 calories, 1 g, 120 mg sodium

tip

If you want to do more vigorous activities, slowly replace those that take moderate effort like brisk walking with more strenuous activities such as jogging. You can add small jogs within your walks and slowly increase the time spent jogging.

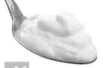

FAST FACT

Frozen yogurt contains probiotic content, which promotes better digestion. Probiotics are good bacteria that can boost your immune system, enhance digestion and even lower cholesterol levels.

YES YOU CAN

Fit in some fat-busting exercises every week. Vigorous-intensity aerobic activity means you're breathing hard and fast, and your heart rate has gone up. Some examples of activities that require vigorous effort: jogging or running, swimming laps, riding a bike fast or on hills, playing singles tennis and playing basketball.

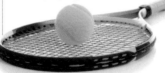

BONUS!

The lactose found in frozen yogurt appears to be more digestible than the lactose in ice cream. Frozen yogurt contains enzymes that assist in breaking down dairy, allowing many people with lactose intolerance to enjoy frozen yogurt with few effects.

ALL YOU! Make sure you're getting enough calcium! Adults between the ages of 19 and 50 need 1,000 mg of calcium per day. Calcium is responsible for developing strong bones and teeth. In addition to dairy products such as milk, yogurt and cottage cheese, great non-dairy sources of calcium include dark leafy greens, broccoli, calcium-fortified soymilk or juices, cereals and beans.

KICK IT

Ben & Jerry's
Chocolate Chip Cookie Dough Ice Cream

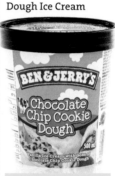

Nutritional Value

SERVING	½ cup
CALORIES	270
FAT	15 g
CARBS	32 g
FIBER	0 g
SUGAR	24 g
SODIUM	85 mg
PROTEIN	4 g

Ditch These Too!

Key lime pie (1 serving)
450 calories, 13 g fat, 240 mg sodium

Regular whipped cream (2 Tbsp)
104 calories, 11.1 g fat, 11 mg sodium

Banana bread (1 slice)
170 calories, 7 g fat, 210 mg sodium

PICK IT

Nutritional Value

SERVING	591 mL
CALORIES	70
FAT	0 g
CARBS	17 g
FIBER	0 g
SUGAR	17 g
SODIUM	270 mg
PROTEIN	0 g

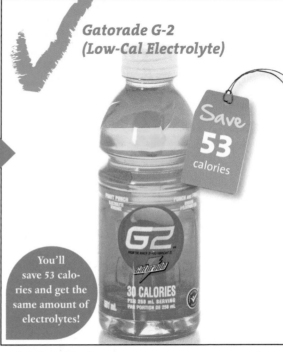

**Gatorade G-2
(Low-Cal Electrolyte)**

Save
53
calories

You'll save 53 calories and get the same amount of electrolytes!

TIP Don't forget your muscles. Cardio won't make you fit all by itself. You should strengthen your muscles at least two days a week. These strengthening activities should work your legs, hips, back, chest, abdomen, shoulders and arms – don't leave any area of your body out! You can strengthen your muscles at home or at the gym.

Give It a Try!

Monster energy drink (low-carb)
10 calories, 0 fat, 180 mg sodium

Diet Rockstar energy drink
10 calories, 0 fat, 146 mg sodium

Sugar-free Red Bull energy drink
10 calories, 0 fat, 204 mg sodium

53

The gallons of carbonated soft drinks and fruit drinks the average American drinks each year. This total exceeds the consumed amounts of milk, fruit juice and bottled water combined.

YES YOU CAN

Try new activities and keep your motivation up at the gym: take a different class, try a water workout such as an aqua fit class or work with a personal trainer for a different perspective.

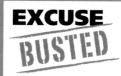

Gatorade Sports Drink (Regular)

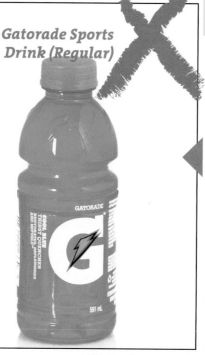

Nutritional Value	
SERVING	591 mL
CALORIES	123
FAT	0 g
CARBS	34.5 g
FIBER	0 g
SUGAR	34.5 g
SODIUM	493 mg
PROTEIN	0 g

EXCUSE
BUSTED

Worried about drinking too much water, so you don't drink enough?

Symptoms of excessive dehydration include nausea, vomiting, muscle weakness, headaches, disorientation and bloating in the face and hands. This is easily avoided. Research suggests that drinking about two cups of water two hours before exercise and another six to eight ounces every 20 minutes can help boost performance.

Ditch These Too!

Monster energy drink (regular)
100 calories, 0 fat, 180 mg sodium

Rockstar energy drink
140 calories, 0 fat, 40 mg sodium

Red Bull energy drink
113 calories, 0 fat, 204 mg sodium

A BETTER CHOICE

Go for whole fruits over fruit juices. Fruit juices may be healthier than soda, but they are also concentrated sources of sugar that don't give you anywhere near the same level of nutrients you get from whole fruits. If you're trying to lose weight, you won't get the same sense of fullness from a glass of juice that you will from a piece of fruit.

PICK IT

Nutritional Value	
SERVING	1 can
CALORIES	50
FAT	0 g
CARBS	10 g
FIBER	2 g
SUGAR	8 g
SODIUM	140 mg
PROTEIN	2 g

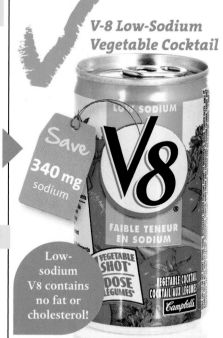

V-8 Low-Sodium Vegetable Cocktail

Save **340 mg** sodium

Low-sodium V8 contains no fat or cholesterol!

BONUS!

V8 is a great source of potassium, which helps manage fluid retention and regulate blood pressure. If you drink one 8-ounce glass of V8 vegetable juice every day, you will have more than your daily requirement for Vitamin A.

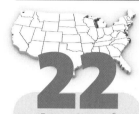

Percentage of American adults who meet recommended physical activity guidelines.

Give It a Try!

Orange juice (1 cup)
121 calories, 0.5 g fat, 3 mg sodium

V8 Splash – strawberry banana (8 oz)
90 calories, 0 fat, 70 mg sodium

Dasani bottled water with lemon
2 calories, 0 fat, 7 mg sodium

>> **FAST FACT**

Eating soy products and cruciferous vegetables, such as cabbage, broccoli and kale can help prevent breast cancer.

Try This

Go for the dark greens. Green vegetables such as kale, broccoli, asparagus and green beans are packed with vitamins A and C, fiber and phytonutrients.

KICK IT

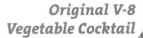

Original V-8 Vegetable Cocktail

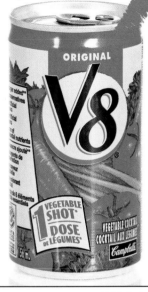

Nutritional Value	
SERVING	1 can
CALORIES	50
FAT	0 g
CARBS	10 g
FIBER	2 g
SUGAR	8 g
SODIUM	480 mg
PROTEIN	2 g

ALL YOU!

Get in that vitamin C! Vitamin C helps your body form collagen (which is the main protein used as connective tissue in the body) in blood vessels, bones, cartilage and muscle. The following foods are good sources of vitamin C: guava, kiwi, strawberries, cantaloupe, papaya, pineapple, mango, raw sweet peppers, Brussels sprouts and, of course, citrus fruits.

Ditch These Too!

Apple cider (8 oz)
120 calories, 0 fat, 25 mg sodium

Lemonade (8 oz)
106 calories, 0.1 g fat, 18 mg sodium

Cream soda (1 can)
189 calories, 0 fat, 45 mg sodium

FATTER, NOT FITTER

Popping a couple of painkillers after a hard workout may seem like a good idea, but a new study suggests these pills do little to relieve post-exercise soreness. What's more, muscle soreness may be a good indicator that you've overextended yourself and that you should ease up a bit on your next workout, rather than just taking a few pills.

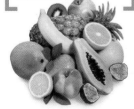

PICK IT

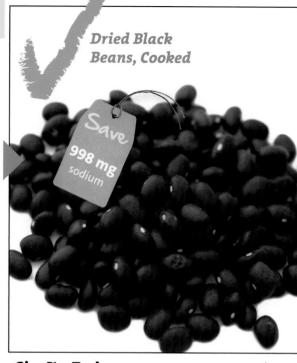

Dried Black Beans, Cooked

Save
998 mg
sodium

A BETTER CHOICE

Canning lowers beans' nutritional value, since they are best lightly cooked for a short period of time, while the canning process cooks them for a long time at higher temperatures.

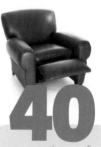

40

percentage of American adults who say they never engage in physical activity during their leisure time.

Give It a Try!

Canned chickpeas (1 cup)
286 calories, 2.6 g fat, 718 mg sodium

Lentils (1 cup)
200 calories, 0.8 g fat, 300 mg sodium

Kidney beans (1 cup)
220 calories, 0.9 g fat, 680 mg sodium

BONUS!

Black beans are a great source of fiber, as are most other legumes. Not only do beans lower cholesterol, but the fiber in black beans also prevents blood sugar levels from rising too rapidly after a meal.

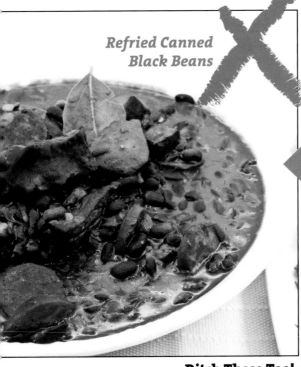

Refried Canned Black Beans

KICK IT

Nutritional Value	
SERVING	½ cup
CALORIES	280
FAT	8 g
CARBS	16 g
FIBER	3 g
SUGAR	0 g
SODIUM	1,000 mg
PROTEIN	4 g

> QUICK & EASY

- Include black beans with other toppings the next time you make a baked potato.

- Soup or chili made with black beans is a great meal or snack option in the winter.

- Blend cooked black beans with tomatoes, onions and your favorite spices to create a delicious bean soup.

Ditch These Too!

Refried pinto beans (1 cup)
237 calories, 3.32 g fat, 753 mg sodium

Canned chili with beans (1 cup)
260 calories, 7 g fat, 1,200 mg sodium

S & W honey mustard baked beans (1 cup)
280 calories, 1 g fat, 1,200 mg sodium

BONUS!

Research published in the *Journal of Agriculture and Food Chemistry* suggests that black beans are as rich as grapes and cranberries in antioxidant compounds called anthocyanins.

INSTANT MEAL COMBO

When combined with whole grains such as brown rice, black beans provide a fat-free complete-protein meal.

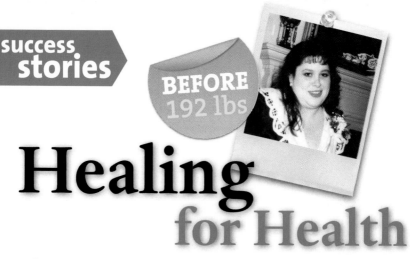

BEFORE
192 lbs

Healing
for Health

After she was sexually abused, Johnna hid behind her extra fat for years, until she finally found the courage to get help and find happiness.

BY WENDY MORLEY

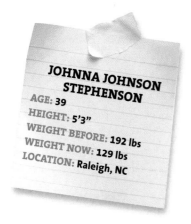

JOHNNA JOHNSON
STEPHENSON
AGE: 39
HEIGHT: 5'3"
WEIGHT BEFORE: 192 lbs
WEIGHT NOW: 129 lbs
LOCATION: Raleigh, NC

"I knew that inside me was a happier, healthier person"

IN HIDING

Johnna didn't realize till much later that her weight gain had come as a direct result of her being sexually abused. Subconsciously, she used extra fat to try and hide her body so no one would notice her. At the age of 28, she confided in a co-worker about what had happened to her and her co-worker convinced her to get therapy. Through therapy, Johnna began to understand that what had happened to her was not her fault. "I knew that inside me was a happier, healthier person," she says. "I started watching what I ate and began an exercise program."

Although she had always struggled with a little excess fat, Johnna kept her weight in check by taking dance classes until her senior year of high school. At that point her weight ballooned and stayed high for the next 10 years.

CONSISTENT DIET IS KEY

Growing up in the South, Johnna was used to eating lots of fried food, but to get healthier she began eating clean – lots of veggies, grilled chicken, apples and raw almonds. Her father always reminded her that success came from long-term consistency, and Johnna says: "He was absolutely right!" She has grown to dislike the fried foods of her youth, preferring clean eats, and if she ever feels tempted she reminds herself of how horrible she feels after eating such foods.

Now a fitness instructor, Johnna incorporates her dance training into her classes. She also trains with weights and says that for her, "exercise has been a lifesaver. I completely love the feeling I get from exercising and lifting weights, which is a huge motivator." Eating correctly has been a bigger challenge, but her recent discovery that she is allergic to wheat has helped her immensely.

HEALTHY AND HAPPY

Health is Johnna's focus now. She doesn't worry about dieting or being skinny. Her meals and snacks are made up of nutritious foods and her habits are healthy. Dancing brings out a feeling of pure joy that leaves her feeling energized and, as she says, "ridiculously happy."

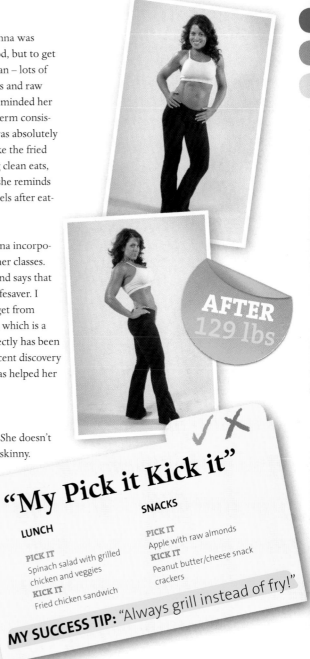

AFTER
129 lbs

✓ ✗

"My Pick it Kick it"

LUNCH

PICK IT
Spinach salad with grilled chicken and veggies

KICK IT
Fried chicken sandwich

SNACKS

PICK IT
Apple with raw almonds

KICK IT
Peanut butter/cheese snack crackers

MY SUCCESS TIP: "Always grill instead of fry!"

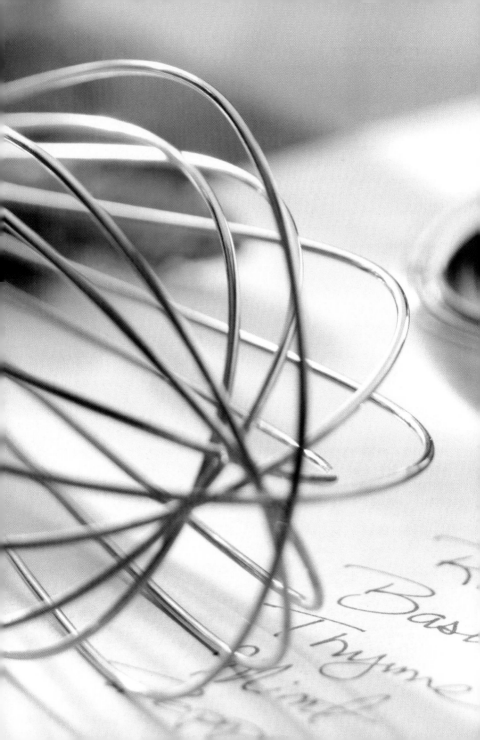

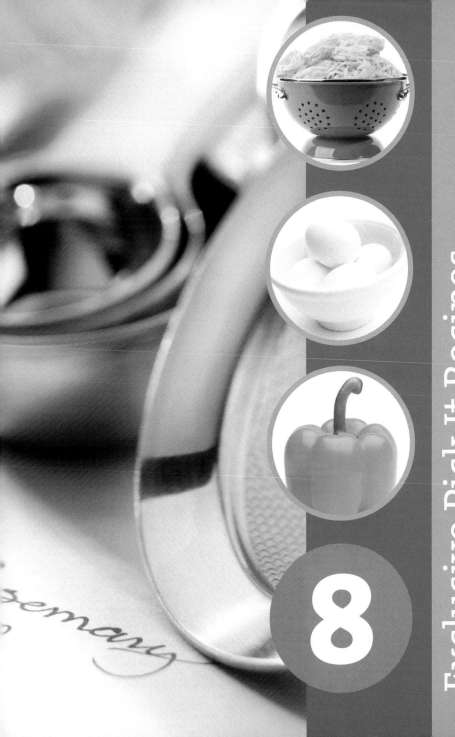

ENERGY BARS

Ready in 30 minutes • Makes 20 servings

1 cup bran flakes cereal

¼ cup each wheat bran and wheat germ

1½ tsp orange peel, grated

¼ cup orange juice

1 cup mixed dried fruit, chopped

1 egg, beaten

¼ cup unsaturated cooking oil

½ cup each applesauce and honey

⅓ cup dry milk powder

¾ cup each whole wheat flour and
   all-purpose flour

¼ tsp baking soda

1. Preheat oven to 350°F. Using some oil, grease a 13" by 9" by 2" pan.

2. In a medium bowl, combine cereal, wheat bran, wheat germ, orange peel, orange juice, dried fruit, egg, oil, applesauce, honey and dry milk powder; blend well. Let set five minutes.

3. In a large bowl, stir together whole wheat flour, all-purpose flour and baking soda. Stir in the first mixture and mix until all ingredients are combined.

4. Spread batter evenly in pan. Bake 15 to 17 minutes or until golden. Cool and serve.

Nutrients per serving:
Calories: 129, Total Fats: 3 g, Saturated Fat: <0.5 g, Cholesterol: 9 mg, Sodium: 79 mg, Total Carbohydrates: 24 g, Dietary Fiber: 2 g, Sugar: 9 g, Protein: 3 g

Quick energy booster!

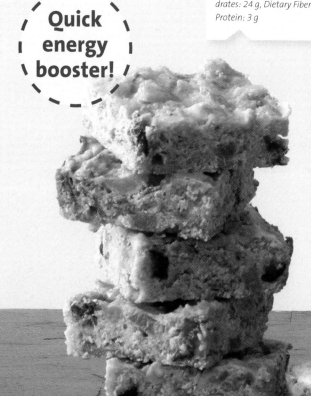

OATMEAL BREAD

Ready in 3 hours • Makes 2 loaves

5¾ to 6¼ cups all-purpose flour, divided

2½ cups old-fashioned oats, uncooked

¼ cup Sucanat

2 x ¼-oz packages (about 4½ teaspoons)
   quick-rising yeast

2½ tsp sea salt

1½ cups water

1¼ cups low-fat milk

4 Tbsp soft tub margarine
   (trans-fat-free type)

Nutrients per 2-slice serving:
Calories: 137, Total Fats: 2 g, Saturated Fat: <0.5 g,
Cholesterol: 1 mg, Sodium: 204 mg, Total Car-
bohydrates: 25 g, Dietary Fiber: 1 g, Sugar: 2 g,
Protein: 4 g

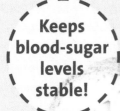

Keeps blood-sugar levels stable!

1. Preheat oven to 375˚F. Grease two loaf pans (8" by 4" or 9" by 5").

2. In a large bowl combine three cups flour, oats, Sucanat, yeast and salt; mix well.

3. In a small saucepan, heat water, milk and margarine until very warm (120˚F to 130˚F). Add to flour mixture. Blend using low speed of electric mixer until dry ingredients are moistened. Increase to medium speed; beat for three minutes. By hand, gradually stir in enough of the remaining flour to make stiff dough.

4. Turn dough out onto lightly floured surface. Knead for five to eight minutes or until smooth and elastic. Shape dough into a ball; place in an oil-greased bowl, turning once. Cover and let rise in a warm place for 30 minutes or until doubled in size.

5. Punch down dough. Cover; let rest 10 minutes. Divide dough in half; shape to form two loaves. Place in two oil-greased loaf pans. Cover and let rise in a warm place for 15 minutes or until nearly doubled in size.

6. Bake at 375˚F for 45 to 50 minutes or until dark golden brown. Remove from pans and place on a wire rack. Cool completely before slicing.

FIT EGGS BENEDICT

Ready in 20 minutes • Makes 2 servings

1 whole grain English muffin, split
2 large, whole eggs
¼ cup nonfat Greek yogurt
2 tsp fresh lemon juice
⅛ tsp powdered mustard
Sea salt, to taste
Dash cayenne pepper
6 asparagus stalks, cooked
Parsley for garnish (optional)

Greek yogurt's high-protein and low-sugar content keeps your appetite at bay.

1. Fill a medium skillet with one inch of water; bring to a boil over medium heat.

2. Meanwhile, toast muffin halves and set aside.

3. When the water reaches a boil, turn the heat down to a simmer, crack one egg at a time into a small dish and gently pour into the simmering water and cook until desired doneness, three to five minutes.

4. While the eggs cook, whisk together yogurt, lemon juice, mustard, salt and cayenne pepper in a small saucepan over low heat; heat until warm—do not boil.

5. To serve, place a toasted muffin on each serving plate and top with three pieces of asparagus. Using a slotted spoon, carefully remove eggs from the water and place one on each muffin; drizzle the yogurt sauce on top of both halves and garnish with parsley. Serve immediately.

Nutrients per serving:
Calories: 170, Total Fat: 6 g, Saturated Fat: 2 g, Trans Fat: 0 g, Cholesterol: 211 mg, Sodium: 363 mg, Total Carbohydrates: 17 g, Dietary Fiber: 3 g, Sugar: 5 g, Protein: 13 g, Iron: 3 mg

Metabolism-boosting brunch!

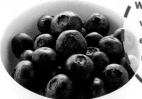

Whole grains provide vitamins and nutrients like fiber, vitamin E, magnesium and potassium.

APPLE-CINNAMON BULGUR

Ready in 30 minutes • Makes 2 servings

¼ cup bulgur (dried cracked wheat)

½ cup low-fat milk

½ cup unsweetened applesauce

1 Tbsp honey

½ tsp cinnamon

¼ tsp nutmeg

½ cup fresh blueberries

2 Tbsp sliced almonds

1. In a small saucepan, combine bulgur and milk; bring to a boil over medium heat. Cover pan tightly and set aside for 25 minutes.

2. Uncover pan and stir in applesauce, honey, cinnamon and nutmeg. Divide into two portions and top each with half the blueberries and almonds; serve immediately.

Nutrients per serving:
Calories: 243, Total Fat: 8 g,
Saturated Fat: 1 g, Trans Fat: 0 g,
Cholesterol: 1 mg, Sodium: 37 mg,
Total Carbohydrates: 41 g, Fiber: 7 g,
Sugar: 22 g, Protein: 8 g, Iron: 1 g

USE NONFAT milk in your post-workout cereal as fat can slow down the muscle-building process by slowing digestion.

ALMONDS can help you maintain a stable blood-sugar level.

SHRIMP, BLACK BEAN AND FETA CHEESE TACOS

Ready in 20 minutes • Makes 4 servings

- 2 Tbsp olive oil, divided
- 2 cups pre-cooked shrimp, shelled
- 2 cups canned black beans, rinsed and drained
- 1 cup salsa
- 4 oz of crumbled low-fat feta cheese
- 8 corn tortillas, 6" diameter
- Avocado slices (optional)

1. Place one Tbsp of olive oil in a large skillet over medium-high heat. Add pre-cooked shrimp and heat until warmed through, about six minutes.

2. Add in black beans and salsa and continue to heat, mixing thoroughly.

3. Cool mixture slightly and add feta cheese.

4. Spoon equal portions into each corn tortilla. Serve with slices of avocado (optional).

Nutrients per serving (without avocado): Calories: 454, Total Fat: 16 g, Saturated Fat: 6 g, Trans Fat: 0 g, Cholesterol: 170 mg, Sodium: 600 mg, Total Carbohydrates: 45 g, Fiber: 8 g, Sugar: 1 g, Protein: 33 g, Iron: 6 mg

Shrimp is a low-fat, low-calorie protein.

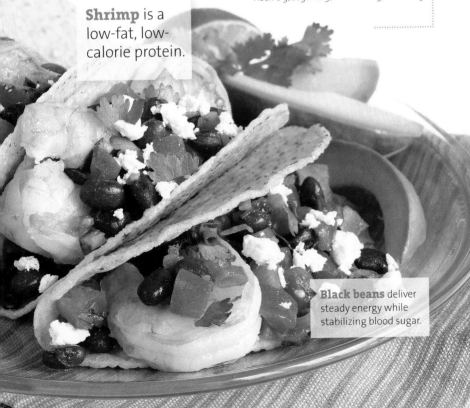

Black beans deliver steady energy while stabilizing blood sugar.

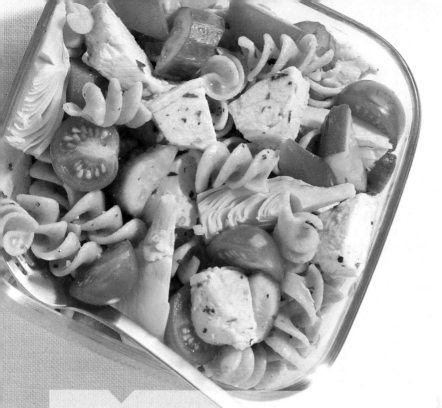

WHOLE WHEAT PASTA SALAD WITH CHICKEN

Ready in 20 minutes • Makes 4 servings

4 chicken breasts (about 1 lb), cooked
   and roughly chopped
8 oz whole wheat pasta, cooked
   and cooled
1 cup cherry tomatoes, halved
½ cucumber, chopped
1 red bell pepper, chopped
4 oz artichoke hearts (reserve
   marinade for dressing)

DRESSING:

1 shallot, minced
1 x 7-oz container Greek yogurt,
   reduced fat (2%)
2 Tbsp reserved marinade

1. In a large bowl, combine chicken,
   pasta, tomatoes, cucumber, pepper
   and artichokes.

2. In a small bowl, combine dressing
   ingredients and stir well. Pour over
   salad.

Nutrients per serving:
Calories: 374, Total Fats: 11 g, Saturated
Fat: 2 g, Trans Fat: 0 g, Cholesterol: 71 mg,
Sodium: 2 mg, Total Carbohydrates: 31 g,
Dietary Fiber: 5 g, Sugar: 7 g, Protein: 36 g,
Iron: 2 mg

GINGER CHICKEN

Ready in 25 minutes • Makes 4 servings

12 oz boneless, skinless
   chicken breasts
½ Tbsp vegetable oil
1 tsp garlic, minced
1 Tbsp fresh ginger, chopped
1 medium onion, cut into wedges
1 large red bell pepper, cut into strips
2 cups broccoli florets
½ cup reduced-sodium chicken broth,
   divided
1 tsp arrowroot powder
2 Tbsp low-sodium soy sauce
2 cups brown rice, cooked and hot

1. Slice chicken breast into bite-size strips. Heat oil in a large skillet over medium-high heat; add chicken and saute for about five minutes. Remove from pan and set aside.

2. Add garlic, ginger, onion, red pepper, broccoli and 1/4 cup chicken broth. Saute until crisp and tender, approximately five minutes.

3. Meanwhile, stir arrowroot powder into the remaining chicken broth and add soy sauce.

4. Return chicken to the pan, add soy sauce mixture and bring to a boil, stirring constantly, until sauce thickens slightly. Cook one minute longer.

5. Serve with brown rice.

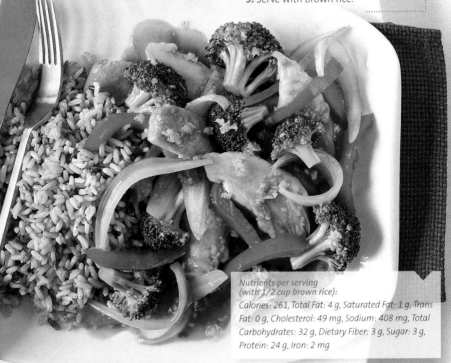

Nutrients per serving
(with 1/2 cup brown rice):
Calories: 261, Total Fat: 4 g, Saturated Fat: 1 g, Trans Fat: 0 g, Cholesterol: 49 mg, Sodium: 408 mg, Total Carbohydrates: 32 g, Dietary Fiber: 3 g, Sugar: 3 g, Protein: 24 g, Iron: 2 mg

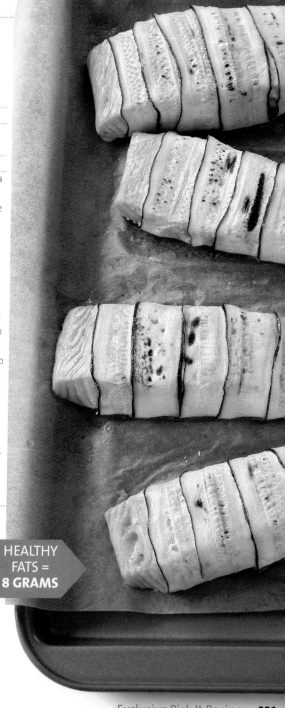

SALMON IN ZUCCHINI CROÛTE

Ready in 15 minutes • Makes 4 servings

2 medium zucchinis

4 salmon fillets (about 1 lb)

Olive oil, sea salt and ground pepper, to taste

1. Preheat broiler to high. Using a vegetable peeler or mandolin slicer, slice zucchini lengthwise into thin strips.

2. Brush salmon fillets with olive oil, salt and pepper to taste. Wrap zucchini around fillets so that the ends are on the bottom, overlapping by about half the width of each zucchini strip. Place on a cookie sheet so that ends are on the bottom, brush a bit more olive oil on top and broil for 10 to 12 minutes.

Nutrients per serving:
Calories: 218, Protein: 24 g, Carbohydrates: 4 g, Fiber: 1 g, Sugar: 2 g, Total Fat: 12 g, Saturated Fat: 4 g, Trans Fat: 0 g, Cholesterol: 57 mg, Sodium: 63 mg, Iron: 1 mg

Lift weights better with essential fats found in fish, which lubricate your joints.

HEALTHY FATS = 8 GRAMS

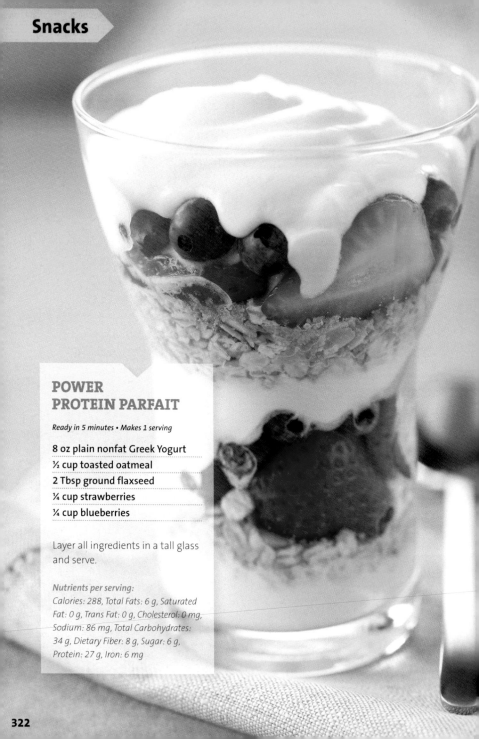

POWER PROTEIN PARFAIT

Ready in 5 minutes • Makes 1 serving

8 oz plain nonfat Greek Yogurt

½ cup toasted oatmeal

2 Tbsp ground flaxseed

¼ cup strawberries

¼ cup blueberries

Layer all ingredients in a tall glass and serve.

Nutrients per serving:
Calories: 288, Total Fats: 6 g, Saturated Fat: 0 g, Trans Fat: 0 g, Cholesterol: 0 mg, Sodium: 86 mg, Total Carbohydrates: 34 g, Dietary Fiber: 8 g, Sugar: 6 g, Protein: 27 g, Iron: 6 mg

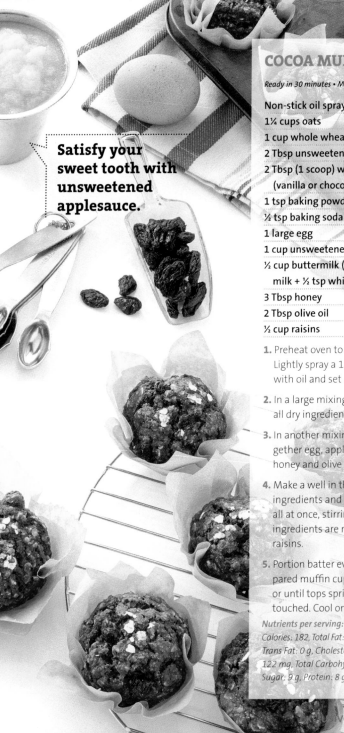

Satisfy your sweet tooth with unsweetened applesauce.

COCOA MUFFINS

Ready in 30 minutes • Makes 12 muffins

Non-stick oil spray

1¼ cups oats

1 cup whole wheat flour

2 Tbsp unsweetened cocoa powder

2 Tbsp (1 scoop) whey protein powder (vanilla or chocolate)

1 tsp baking powder

½ tsp baking soda

1 large egg

1 cup unsweetened applesauce

½ cup buttermilk (or ½ cup low-fat milk + ½ tsp white vinegar)

3 Tbsp honey

2 Tbsp olive oil

½ cup raisins

1. Preheat oven to 350°F degrees. Lightly spray a 12-cup muffin pan with oil and set aside.

2. In a large mixing bowl, combine all dry ingredients.

3. In another mixing bowl, whisk together egg, applesauce, buttermilk, honey and olive oil.

4. Make a well in the center of the dry ingredients and pour in egg mixture all at once, stirring just until all dry ingredients are moistened. Stir in raisins.

5. Portion batter evenly into the prepared muffin cups. Bake 20 minutes or until tops spring back when lightly touched. Cool on a wire rack.

Nutrients per serving:
Calories: 182, Total Fat: 4 g, Saturated Fat: 1 g, Trans Fat: 0 g, Cholesterol: 20 mg, Sodium: 122 mg, Total Carbohydrates: 30 g, Fiber: 4 g, Sugar: 9 g, Protein: 8 g, Iron: 2 mg

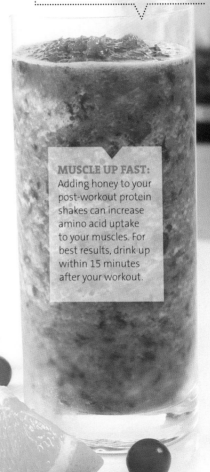

CRANBERRY PROTEIN SHAKE

Ready in 10 minutes • Makes 2 servings

- 1 cup fresh or frozen cranberries, rinsed and drained
- 1 medium orange, peeled and coarsely chopped
- 1 cup freshly squeezed orange juice
- 2 scoops plain or vanilla whey protein powder
- 1 tsp honey, optional

Place all ingredients in a blender and process until smooth. Serve immediately over ice.

Nutrients per serving:
Calories: 191, Total Fats: 0 g, Saturated Fat: 0 g, Trans Fat: 0 g, Cholesterol 10 mg, Sodium: 77 mg, Total Carbohydrates: 28 g, Dietary Fiber: 4 g, Sugar: 21 g, Protein: 19 g, Iron: 2 mg

MUSCLE UP FAST: Adding honey to your post-workout protein shakes can increase amino acid uptake to your muscles. For best results, drink up within 15 minutes after your workout.

WHEY ALL THE WAY: Not only is it the fastest digesting type of protein, but whey also has the most branched-chain amino acids, critical for muscle growth.

STAY SLIM: One cup of cranberries has only 44 calories, is high in fiber and low in sugar.

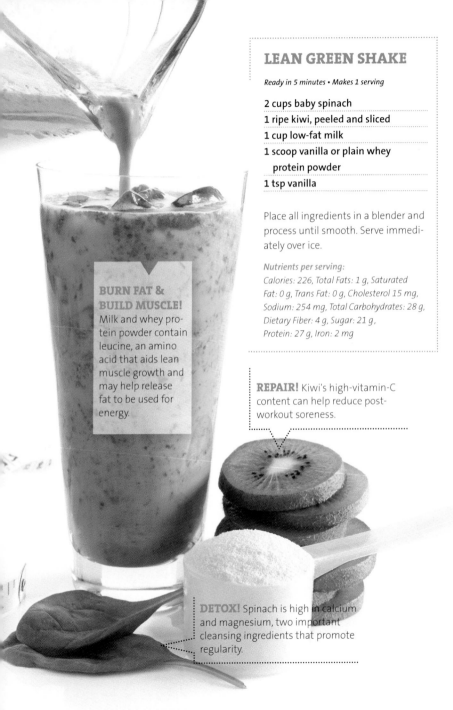

LEAN GREEN SHAKE

Ready in 5 minutes • Makes 1 serving

2 cups baby spinach

1 ripe kiwi, peeled and sliced

1 cup low-fat milk

1 scoop vanilla or plain whey protein powder

1 tsp vanilla

Place all ingredients in a blender and process until smooth. Serve immediately over ice.

Nutrients per serving:
Calories: 226, Total Fats: 1 g, Saturated Fat: 0 g, Trans Fat: 0 g, Cholesterol 15 mg, Sodium: 254 mg, Total Carbohydrates: 28 g, Dietary Fiber: 4 g, Sugar: 21 g, Protein: 27 g, Iron: 2 mg

BURN FAT & BUILD MUSCLE! Milk and whey protein powder contain leucine, an amino acid that aids lean muscle growth and may help release fat to be used for energy.

REPAIR! Kiwi's high-vitamin-C content can help reduce post-workout soreness.

DETOX! Spinach is high in calcium and magnesium, two important cleansing ingredients that promote regularity.

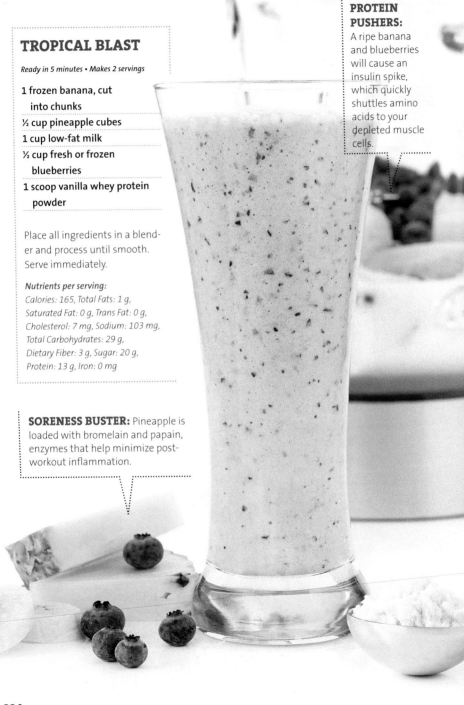

TROPICAL BLAST

Ready in 5 minutes • Makes 2 servings

1 frozen banana, cut into chunks
½ cup pineapple cubes
1 cup low-fat milk
½ cup fresh or frozen blueberries
1 scoop vanilla whey protein powder

Place all ingredients in a blender and process until smooth. Serve immediately.

Nutrients per serving:
Calories: 165, Total Fats: 1 g,
Saturated Fat: 0 g, Trans Fat: 0 g,
Cholesterol: 7 mg, Sodium: 103 mg,
Total Carbohydrates: 29 g,
Dietary Fiber: 3 g, Sugar: 20 g,
Protein: 13 g, Iron: 0 mg

SORENESS BUSTER: Pineapple is loaded with bromelain and papain, enzymes that help minimize post-workout inflammation.

PROTEIN PUSHERS: A ripe banana and blueberries will cause an insulin spike, which quickly shuttles amino acids to your depleted muscle cells.

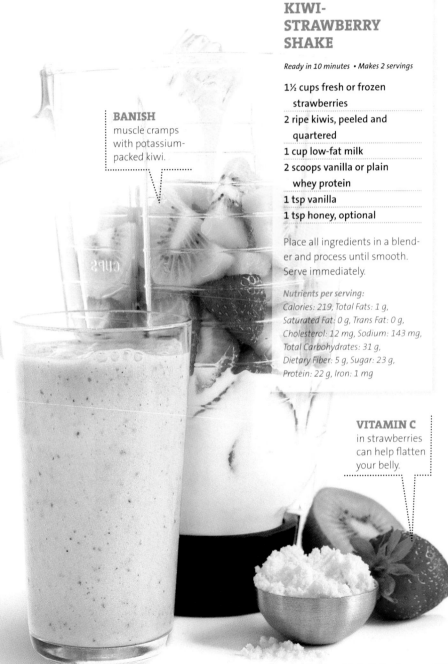

KIWI-STRAWBERRY SHAKE

Ready in 10 minutes • Makes 2 servings

1½ cups fresh or frozen strawberries

2 ripe kiwis, peeled and quartered

1 cup low-fat milk

2 scoops vanilla or plain whey protein

1 tsp vanilla

1 tsp honey, optional

Place all ingredients in a blender and process until smooth. Serve immediately.

Nutrients per serving:
Calories: 219, Total Fats: 1 g,
Saturated Fat: 0 g, Trans Fat: 0 g,
Cholesterol: 12 mg, Sodium: 143 mg,
Total Carbohydrates: 31 g,
Dietary Fiber: 5 g, Sugar: 23 g,
Protein: 22 g, Iron: 1 mg

BANISH
muscle cramps with potassium-packed kiwi.

VITAMIN C
in strawberries can help flatten your belly.

123RF: 127 (fish and chips), 169 (nutrition label), 287 (tea bag)

Baker, Rich: Cover (hand model Samantha Israel), 12, 22 (Shredded Wheat), 23 (Oatmeal Crisp), 28 (Quaker Oats), 29 (Quaker Oatmeal), 36-37, 64-65, 67 (sandwich), 155-157 (product shots), 164-167 (product shots), 235, 240 (Amy's Organic Chili), 258 (rice vinegar), 260-261 (product shots), 264-265, 267 (Orville Redenbacher's), 270-275 (product shots), 288-289, 298-299, 302-307 (product shots); prop styling by Jessica Pensabene, Brian Ross and Ellie Jeon

Beaven, Pat: 175 (Meagan Hesham)

Big Stock: Sweet potatoe fries (cover, 46, 226)

Bradshaw, Doug: 322

Bucetta, Paul: Back cover (Diane Hart), 58-59 (pizza), 66, 72-75 (Taco Bell products), 137, 173, 206-207 (pantry), 209-211 (pantry), 232-233 (Smart Water, Crystal Light)

Cherry-go-round: 154

Chou, Peter: 7 (tacos), 53 (shrimp salad), 54-55 (food stylist Claire Stubbs, prop sylist Catherine Doherty), 195 (flank steak), 252-256, 316-321, 323

Crank, Rick: 311 (Johnna Stephenson)

Elliot, Brandon C.: 141 (Tammy Stewart)

Gibson & Smith: 56-57 (food stylist Marianne Wren), 63 (tuna and sushi), 68-71 (food stylist Terry Schacht, prop stylist Catherine Doherty), 102, 187 (ratatouille)

Guzman, Gabriel: 91 (Beth Peshia)

Henderson, Joey: 247 (Miranda Henderson)

Jupiter Images: 54 (salad bar), 138-139 (kitchen)

Kushniryk, Katelynn: 41 (Nicole Sampson)

Pensabene, Jessica: Cover (foot model Stephanie Pereira)

Pond, Edward: 31 (background), 32-33, 314-315

Quaker Oats Company: 170 (Quaker Quakes), 172 (rice cakes)

Reiff, Robert: 86-87 (chicken & white bean soup)

Salinas, Andrea: 205 (Allison Earnst)

Stoneyfield Farms: 150

Veer: 8-9 (orange), 286

Visnyei, Maya: 7 (shake), 144, 324-327

All other photos from **iStockphoto.com**.

Acknowledgments

This book is the result of several months of work on the part of many people who make *Oxygen* magazine the top fitness and health source for women.

First, I'd like to thank Robert Kennedy for giving me the opportunity to undertake this project and guide it with his unique vision and drive, and his wife Tosca Reno, *Oxygen* columnist and best-selling author of *The Eat-Clean Diet®* series, for her un-wavering support and encouragement; to all the staff at Robert Kennedy Publishing whose help I requested from time to time – sometimes with my customary "energy" – and who never turned me down no matter the crushing deadlines they faced.

Special thanks to the book team at Robert Kennedy Publishing, especially Jessica Pensabene, acting art director, who tackled a complex, challenging project with a smile and Wendy Morley, who managed to work magic with high-tech-editing tools. (Gotta love those scissors!)

In particular I'd like to thank the staff and contributors at *Oxygen* and *Clean Eating* magazines, many of whom found time in their busy schedules to hunt down second-ary research or nutritional information, and *Oxygen*'s art director Stacy Jarvis, whose contributions in the final stages of this book have proven invaluable. My grateful thanks to the entire art, editorial and production team at *Oxygen* and *Clean Eating* magazines – you've all contributed to this project in some way and I thank you very much. I'd like to thank the many writers and photographers I'm privileged to work with, as well as the nutritionists, regular contributors, exercise physiologists and fitness experts, all of whom make *Oxygen* the magazine it is – the unparalleled leader in women's fitness.

In addition, I'd like to thank my daughter Kate for her generous – and timely – offer of additional research and writing, and to my son Drew for his unstinting support throughout the months, in person and in emails and texts from his travels here and abroad.

Finally, I'd like to thank Jerry Kindela, Robert Kennedy Publishing's group editorial director, for agreeing to take on this dense project along with his many responsibilities and do with it what he does best – make things happen.

- Diane

INDEX

A

A Healthy Breakfast, 30
alcohol, 149, 184
allicin, 235
almonds, 26-27, 153, 317
Alzheimer's disease, 182-183
American Dietetic Association, 77-78, 128, 240, 254
American Heart Association, 13, 253, 272, 275, 277, 291
American Journal of Clinical Nutrition, 127, 224
antioxidants, 101, 106, 188-189, 217, 273
Appetite, 59, 145, 237
apple, 237
   Apple-Cinnamon Bulgur, 317
applesauce, 236-237, 314, 317, 323
Arby's, 180
Archives of Internal Medicine, 81
avocado, 76-77
avocado oil, 57
Avocado Oil & Vinegar Dressing, 57

B

bacon, 34-35
bagel, 38-39
balance, 274
Barnard, Dr. Neal, 125

BBQ Chicken Pita Pocket, 70
beans, 49, 74, 87, 240, 308-309
   Shrimp, Black Bean and Feta Cheese Tacos, 318
Beasley, Tammy, 39
Ben & Jerry's, 302-303
berries, mixed, 23
Birds Eye, 128
bisphenol-A (BPA), 129, 263
blood pressure, 255
BMI (Body Mass Index), 60
Bob Evans, 181
bread, 68, 84-85
   Ezekiel, 69
   Oatmeal Bread, 315
   rye, 71
breakfast, 11, 19, 182, 260
breast cancer, 130
British Journal of Nutrition, 11, 289
British Medical Journal, 255
broccoli, 106-107
buffet, 199
Burger King, 182
Bust Fat With Your Groceries, 210-213

C

cabbage, 221
caffeine, 15, 294-295
calcium, 64, 151, 171, 224

calories, 11, 135, 199
   cutting, 160-161
Campbell's soups, 88-89
Cancer Research, 221
candy, 149
canned meals, 240-241
cabohydrates (carbs), 85, 191
Carl's Jr., 183
carotenoids, 183, 213
cataracts, 50
celery, 86
cereal, 260-261
cheese,
   Cheese Scramble Sandwich, 257
   dip, 60-61
   ricotta, 120
   Shrimp, Black Bean and Feta Cheese Tacos, 318
   snacks, 170-171
Cheese Scramble Sandwich, 257
chicken, 100-101, 110, 114-115, 183, 190, 228
   BBQ Chicken Pita Pocket, 70
   canned, 82
   Chicken Curry, 256
   Ginger Chicken, 320
   skin, 114
   Whole-Wheat Pasta Salad With Chicken, 319
Chicken Curry, 256

chickpeas, 80-81
chili, 104-105, 240-241
Chili's, 184
Chinese food, 202
chips, 147, 164-165, 170-171, 228, 298-299
chocolate, 148-149, 153, 172-173, 272-275
cholesterol, 27, 149
Chunky soups, 89
cinnamon, 17
Clark, Nancy, 13
Classico, 216
Clean Eating, 205
Clinical Nutrition, 290
cocoa, 264
  Cocoa Muffins, 323
condiments, 214-215, 220-225, 238-239
corn, 128-129, 188
crackers, 146-147, 230-231
Cranberry Protein Shake, 324
cravings, 65, 70, 172, 187
cupboards, 212-213
cutting boards, 139

D

dairy, 12, 30, 116, 120, 281-283
deep breathing, 66
Deli Salad, 257
Denny's, 185
diabetes, 23, 113, 185
diet, low-carb, 128
Diet Detective's Countdown, The, 179

dieting, 18, 25
Digate Muth, Natalie, 99
digestive process, 119
dogs, 61
Domino's pizza, 186
Doritos, 170-171
drinks, 228, 268
  caffeinated, 15, 294-295
  caloric, 169
  diet, 148
  dinner, 98
  energy, 287
  sports, 163, 304-305
Drop Pounds Easily, 160-161
durum wheat, 31

E

Earnst, Allison, 204-205
Eason, Jamie, 204
Easy Dinnertime Fat Loss, 94-95
Eat-Clean Diet®, The, 204, 247
eating,
  basics, 138
  colors, 164, 183, 262
  companion, 59
  Eating Out?, 200
  frequency, 105
  habits, 62-63, 75, 79, 94-95, 108, 167, 192
  Mindful Eating, 118-119
  quickly, 198
Eating Out?, 200
eggs, 20-21, 30, 229
  Fit Eggs Benedict, 316
energy,
  bar, 264-265

Energy Bars, 314
  foods, 296
  snacks, 297
Energy Bars, 314
Engel, Kathleen, 204-205
Enjoy The Journey!, 174
estrogen, 125
ethnic foods, 202-203
European Journal of Clinical Nutrition, 295
exercise, 195, 265, 269, 279, 283, 303

F

fat, 277
  healthy, 77, 146
  loss, 20, 29, 31, 63, trans fat, 146-147, 275
fiber, 81, 220, 271
fish, 98-99, 126-127, 227, 321
Fit Eggs Benedict, 316
Five Great Healthy Kitchen Gadgets, 139
flavor, 172
folate, 188
Food Rules: An Eater's Manual, 163
Foods For More Energy, 296
fries, 46-47
frozen snacks, 270-271, 302-303
fruit, 162, 227, 229
  juice, 163, 229, 232-233, 290-291
  snacks, 154-155
frying, deep, 47

G

garlic, 187, 234-235
Gatorade, 304-305
Ginger Chicken, 320
Glaceau Smartwater, 232
glutathione, 106
gluten, 31
glycemic index, 237
Go Ahead, Have A Snack, 144-145
goals, 46
grains, whole, 13, 31, 124, 133, 157, 213, 229, 260
grapefruit, 35
grater/zester, 139
Green Giant, 128-129
grocery shopping, 134, 211

H

Häagen-Dazs, 150-151
Hamburger Helper, 134-135
Healing for Health, 310-311
heart disease, 255-256
Henderson, Miranda, 246-247
Herbed Lentils, 254
Hesham, Meagan, 174-175
high fructose corn syrup, 156
horseradish, 222-223
hot flashes, 193
human growth hormone (HGH), 29
hydration, 193, 284
hypertension, 250

I

"I Did it On My Own," 40-41
ice cream, 151
immunity, 255
insulin, 48, 255
International Journal of Obesity, 25
iodine, 21
iron, 180, 243
Is Your Salad Making You Fat?, 54-55
Italian food, 202

J

Jack In The Box, 186
Jamieson-Petonic, Amy, 11
Japanese food, 203
Jerk Fish, 253
Johnson Stephenson, Johnna, 310-311
journal, food, 122
Journal of Agriculture and Food Chemistry, 287, 309
Journal of Nutrition, 17, 26, 225

K

Kashi, 156-157, 230
Keep In Mind, 201
kefir, 280-281
Kellogg's, 36-37
Ketteler, Judi, 246-247
KFC, 188
kiwi,
    Kiwi-Strawberry Shake, 327

Lean Green Shake, 325
Know Your Oats, 32-33

L

labels, 232
lactose, 303
Lakatos, Lyssie, 253
Larsen, Jamie, 27
Lay's, 165
Lean Green Shake, 325
Lean Up Your Lunch!, 44-45
leftovers, 137
lemon, 238-239
leucine, 325
light foods, 45, 267
Long John Silver's, 189
lunch, 65
lycopene, 217

M

magnesium, 65, 193
Marie Callender's, 130-131
marinades, 238-239
massage, 103
McDonald's, 14-15, 64-65, 167, 190
meals,
    canned, 240-241
    energy, 297
    restaurant, 96
    skipping, 34
meat, 278-279
    beef, 195
    chicken, 100-101, 110, 114-115, 183, 190, 228
    deli, 78-79
        Deli Salad, 257

ground, 135
portions, 123
red, 35, 131
roast, 130-131
steak, 108-109
turkey, 35, 122, 135, 278
Menopause, 193
mental clarity, 24
menu, self-care, 180
metabolism, 75, 255
Mexican food, 203
Meyers, Stephanie, 119
Michelina's, 132-133
milk, 165, 229, 292-293, 317
Mindful Eating, 118-119
Moloo, Jeannie, 254-255
Morley, Wendy, 90-91, 140-141, 174-175, 310-311
muffins, 14-15, 24-25
Cocoa Muffins, 323
multigrain, 84
mustard, 79
Honey Dijon Dressing, 57

N

Nabisco, 146-147
Nancy Clark's Sports Nutrition Guidebook, 13
National Weight Control Registry, 11
New England Journal of Medicine, 111
New York City, 67
New York Times, The, 95, 232
niacin, 114, 183
"No More Excuses!", 90-91

No-Salt, Lowest Sodium Cookbook, The, 254
Nutri-Grain bar, 157
nutrients, 190
Nutrients To Keep You Lean, 276
nutrition, 181
Nutrition & Metabolism, 120
Nutrition Journal, 60
nuts, 26-27, 228, 300-301

O

oatmeal, 16-17, 28-29, 227
Oatmeal Bread, 315
oats, 31-33
Obama, Michelle, 216
obese, 111
Obesity, 38, 61
oil, 212, 229
Avocado Oil and Vinegar Dressing, 57
Flaxseed Oil Dressing, 57
sprayer, 139
Olive Garden, 191
omega-3 fatty acids, 127, 277
orange, 162-163
juice, 12, 163, 197, 288-289
Orange Poppy Seed Dressing, 56
osteoporosis, 121
Outback Steakhouse, 192
overindulging, 178
Oxygen, 40, 54, 118, 204-205, 205, 209, 247
Oxygen cooler, 51

P

pantry, 138, 212-213
pasta, 120-121, 132-133
Pasta Primavera, 132
Whole-Wheat Pasta Salad With Chicken, 319
pearl barley, 213
peppers, chili, 104
Perky, Henry Drushel, 261
Peshia, Beth, 90-91
pineapple, 326
pistachios, 158, 266-267
pita, whole wheat, 70
pizza, 58-59, 96-97
Pizza Hut, 58-59
Planters, 154-155, 158-159
plastic, 70
Platkin, Charles Stuart, 179
Pollan, Michael, 163
pomegranate juice, 290
popcorn, 148-149
Popeye's, 193
portions, 185, 198, 209, 211
potassium, 285
potatoes, 46-47, 77, 116-117, 226
baked, 112-113
scalloped, 116-117
Power Protein Parfait, 322
President Barack Obama, 121
Pringles, 164-165
probiotics, 244
protein, 11, 20, 74-75, 99, 190
Cranberry Protein Shake, 324

Power Protein Parfait, 322

shakes, 36

sources, 30

soy, 69

whey, 324

pumpkin, 213

Q

Quaker, 28-29

R

refrigerator, 138

Reno, Tosca, 118, 247

rest, 109

restaurants, 96, 111, 200-201

rice, 124-125

rice cookers, 139

Roast Beef On Sourdough, 68

Rolls, Barbara, 145

S

salad, 44-45, 48-49, 100-101

Deli Salad, 257

dressing, 50-53, 214-215

Avocado Oil &
Vinegar, 57

Flaxseed Oil, 57

Honey Dijon, 57

Orange Poppy
Seed, 56

Soy Ginger
Sesame, 56

Two Minutes
To Your Best
Homemade
Dressing, 56

Is Your Salad Making
You Fat?, 54-55

spinner, 139

Whole Wheat Pasta
Salad With
Chicken, 319

salmon, 71, 98, 189, 213

Salmon BLT on Rye, 71

Salmon in Zucchini
Croute, 321

salsa, 192, 218-219

salt, 67, 73, 250-255

Sampson, Nicole, 40-41

sandwiches, 68-71

BBQ Chicken Pita
Pocket, 70

Roast Beef On
Sourdough, 68

Salmon BLT on Rye, 71

Turkey Caesar On
Ezekiel, 69

sauces, 216-217

sauerkraut, 220

sausage, 122-123

seafood, 98-99, 127

Secret to Skinny, The, 253

selenium, 122

sensory-specific satiety, 56

Shake Your Salt Habit,
250-256

Shape Up Your Kitchen,
208-209

shrimp, 98-99

Shrimp, Black Bean and
Feta Cheese Tacos, 318

Shredded Wheat, 261

sinks, 136

skin, 154

Slash Calories, 10-11

sleep, 29

snack bars, 156-157

snacking, 145

soda, 145, 228

sodium, 147, 158-159, 250-257, 259

soup, 86-89, 227

Soup's On!, 86-87

soy sauce, 258-259

Soy Ginger Sesame
Dressing, 56

spinach, 87, 242-243

spreads, 12-13, 26-27, 80-81

stability ball, 61

steak, 108-109

steamer basket, 139

steps, 84-85

Stewart, Tammy, 140-141

Stoynev, Jennifer, 14

strength training, 195, 272

stress, 70, 104

Subway, 66-67, 194

Success Stories

Earnst, Allison, 204-205

Henderson, Miranda,
246-247

Hesham, Meagan, 174-175

Johnson Stephenson,
Johnna, 310-311

Peshia, Beth, 90-91

Sampson, Nicole, 40-41

Stewart, Tammy, 140-141

Sudden Impact, 246-247

sugar, 170, 273

sunflower seeds, 52

sushi, 103

sweeteners, artificial, 198

T

Taco Bell, 72-75, 194
tea,
  chamomile, 286-287
  green, 14, 294-295
tempura, 63
Thayer, Beth, 240
This Mom Looks Better
  Than Ever!, 140-141
tilapia, 191
tomatoes, 216-217
tooth enamel decay, 145
Top 5 Energy Snacks, 297
Trader Joe's, 24-25
training partner, 97
triglycerides, 71
Tropical Blast, 326
tuna, 82-83, 127
  Tuna Pita, 257
  Tuna Roll, 102-103
turkey, 35, 122, 135, 278
  Turkey Caesar On
    Ezekiel, 69
  Turkey Wrap, 257
turmeric, 256
TV, 46
Two Minutes To Your Best
  Homemade Dressing, 56

U

V

V-8, 306-307
Van Den Broek, Astrid,
  40-41
vegetables, 187, 220, 228,
  262-263

leafy greens, 242-243
vinegar,
  Avocado Oil & Vinegar,
    57
  balsamic, 214-215
  rice wine, 258-259
visualization, 50
vitamin B-12, 270
vitamin B6, 183
vitamin C, 289, 307
vitamins, 181
Volumetrics Eating Plan, The,
  145

W

waist size, 13, 72
walking, 267-269
water, 38, 233, 284-285
  flavored, 232-233
weight loss, 20, 29, 31, 63,
  160-161
Wendy's, 166
White, Jim, 128
White Bean Dip, 231
Whole Wheat Pasta Salad
  With Chicken, 319
wine, 99
workout, 74, 109, 169, 172,
  287, 293
  morning, 11
  program, 181

X

Y

yogurt, 18-19, 224-225, 227,
  244
  frozen, 150, 302-303
  Greek, 282, 316
Young, Lisa, 197
Young, Meredith, 59
Your 3 Pantry Must-Haves,
  213
Your Fast/Food Guide,
  178-179
Your Guide to the Best
  Oats, 31
Your Pick It Kick It Kitchen,
  136-139
Your Restaurant Survival
  Guide, 196-199
Your Top 15, 226-229

Z

OTHER TITLES FROM ROBERT KENNEDY PUBLISHING

THE EAT-CLEAN DIET® RECHARGED!   BESTSELLER

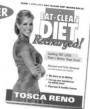

The original *Eat-Clean Diet®* helped readers understand how to get lean and stay healthy forever. Three years later, hundreds of thousands of people have overcome their weight and health problems by following Tosca Reno's Eat-Clean lifestyle. This larger, totally redesigned, revised and fully updated edition offers more in-depth information on non-threatening exercise, staying motivated, banishing cellulite and loose skin, extending and improving your life, and much more! Also includes 50 new recipes and brand-new meal plans!

THE EAT-CLEAN DIET® COOKBOOK   BESTSELLER

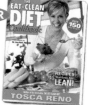

A perfect follow-up, this best-selling cookbook is bound to be your go-to guide for Clean meals, with over 150 recipes and gorgeous color photos throughout. From soups and sauces to main courses and desserts, Tosca touches on every food group, combining them into easy-to-prepare, delicious meals that are crowd favorites. Bonus info pages explain the Eat-Clean Principles, protein facts, sugar substitutes and more. Grab your apron and heat up the oven because delicious, healthy food is on the menu tonight!

THE EAT-CLEAN DIET® FOR FAMILY & KIDS

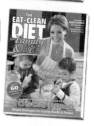

Tosca Reno has changed the face of health, diet and fitness with her Eat-Clean revolution, and now she's delivering that message to the family. In her foreword, cosmetics icon, CEO and mother-of-three Bobbi Brown says, "Tosca Reno's newest book could not have come at a better time ... Healthy eating needs to start at home and it is our obligation as parents to set the right example for our kids." With tons of tips, tricks and advice, in addition to 60 kid-friendly recipes, this book is sure to become your biggest resource.

TOSCA RENO'S EAT CLEAN COOKBOOK   BESTSELLER

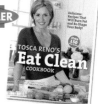

Taste and health come together at last in Tosca Reno's kitchen. Accompanied by bright, colorful photographs by renowned food photographer Donna Griffith, Tosca gives you 150 brand-new mouth-watering recipes, designed with your waistline and palate in mind. In her meals, which are quick to prepare and easy to enjoy, Tosca pairs local cuisine with exotic flavors, giving seasoned chefs and cooking novices alike delectable recipes that everyone will love.

OXYGEN NO PAIN NO GAIN TRAINING JOURNAL

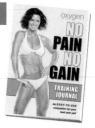

Meet your fitness and health goals with this personal motivator and resource tool in one. The *Oxygen No Pain No Gain Training Journal* provides weight-training newcomers and seasoned fitness buffs alike with a convenient, easy-to-use and self-explanatory tracking system that makes it a cinch to follow workout progress over time. Includes daily training journal pages with a place to note weight and reps for up to 15 different exercises, as well space for cardio notes and goals.

For even more book titles by Robert Kennedy Publishing, please visit rkpubs.com

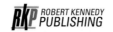

ROBERT KENNEDY
PUBLISHING